Training for Mass

Gordon LaVelle

Romanart Books

This book is dedicated to everyone who helped make its first printing a success--and to all the photographers who declared that no one would ever buy a bodybuilding book that didn't have pictures.

Consult a physician before beginning any exercise program.

www.trainingformass.com

Contents

Contents

Prologue

This is not a typical workout book. One obvious difference between this and nearly all other works of its type is the absence of pictures. In this book, there are none. Traditionally, workout books are filled with them, as this is often seen as a major selling point. These books will enlist the images of current or recent top bodybuilders, either performing exercises or merely showing their muscles, or even eating. The idea is that the association of these images will validate the ideas presented in the sometimes sparse and often simplistic text with which they are mingled. In fact, these books tend to advertise the models displayed in the hundreds of photos as much as the routines and concepts they outline. The association of the images, readily apparent to the potential buyer leafing through the pages in the bookstore, is meant to suggest that the ideas presented therein will allow one to emulate these bodybuilders—much as a cookbook will have fantastic shots of elegantly prepared meals. In the case of each, it is suggested that if you follow the accompanying instructions, here will be the result. It only takes a few seconds of looking at a picture to appreciate that a meal had been elegantly prepared, or that a bodybuilder had built a world-class physique.

I have read quite a few of these books. They all seem to attempt to elicit a visual impact, but their ideas are often suspect, or blasé, or in many cases just wrong. The concepts presented are typically secondary or of little consequence to the purpose of the book. Not all workout books fall into this category, as some go to lengths to discuss the logic behind the strategies they prescribe. But these are few in number. Most are not worth reading.

Many are the gratuitous offerings of established bodybuilders, who are always looking for something to sell alongside their videos, signed photos, and signature-line food supplements and clothing. All of this being considered, who cares what they say? Their primary purpose is to cash in on the imagery or the fame the author, not impart useful information or uncover the truth.

The desire to impart useful information and attempting to uncover the truth are central to the purpose of this book. This is what makes this book valuable, not a large collection of pictures. Incorporating such a collection is somewhat insulting to the intelligence of the reader anyway; it is as if he is being told that the ideas *must* be valid, as evidenced by the photos accompanying the text. Weight training to increase muscle mass, and indeed physical performance in general, can be discussed as a serious topic. I have approached much of this subject from a philosophical perspective—and as most people would be able to tell you, few books on that topic are crammed with pictures.

And why would anyone who wants to look at bodybuilders buy a book to accomplish this? There are limitless numbers of pictures free for the viewing on the internet, more than one could spend a lifetime perusing. Magazines have huge numbers of pictures as well, and the subscriptions are cheap. A years' subscription to one of the major titles might cost little more than the price of many of the training books currently on the market. Buy one, and each month you will get lots and lots of new pictures to examine. In this regard, no book can compete.

It is true that bodybuilding is a physical pursuit, with physical execution as the vehicle for its accomplishment. Inasmuch, nearly all these books have pictures depicting bodybuilders performing the exercises. This book assumes that the reader knows how a certain exercise is performed. If he doesn't, it is not advisable to induce this information by looking at pictures. He should get a trainer, a good one, to show him correct form. And again, often times the pictures of exercise execution seem little more than advertisements for the models depicted.

In this respect this book is different. Granted, there is a picture of me on the back cover, which would seem to contradict my statements regarding the association of imagery and information. The picture is there because I am the author; and though pretty understated, it also implies to some degree that I practice what I preach, and that the ideas presented in this book have merit—at least insofar as they are capable of producing results. I have, in fact, built a good deal of muscle. There are more pictures on my website if anyone has doubts.

But quite beyond this, I have gone to lengths to show that the concepts in the book are theoretically sound. I am definitely not, however, an armchair theorist. I have spent a great many years "in the trenches" using the exact methods conveyed by this book. And this is a point of no small consequence, because much of the information in this book contradicts prevailing views of exercise science. And yes, even in the seemingly rudimentary world of weight training, there is theoretical controversy. Several of the ideas in this book are not of my own invention, and I give credit where credit is due. In these cases, I have merely tried to provide a concise explanation of what others have postulated; where appropriate, I have introduced my own opinions based on personal experience or observation, or logical consideration.

So what is left is text. This book has ideas, lots of them. This is the value I have to bring to the topic. I am a bodybuilder, but I am not a famous one, so the importance of this book has to be in its perspective. If I did not believe that I had original and valuable ideas to convey, I never would have written it. Nor are my ideas commercially conceived. I do not support or recommend any commercial ventures that have anything to do with the bodybuilding or the fitness industries. I have no income whatsoever that is related to these industries. I have no affiliations. But I have a logical mind, a skeptical outlook, and a desire to uncover the truth. I also have (as of this printing) more than a quarter-century of experience. And I have been successful. At the same time, I will not pretend that the importance of personal experience exceeds the value of rational inquiry. Everything in the Universe is amenable to scientific examination, and weight training for the purpose of building mass is no exception.

I

The Problem

Anything worth doing is worth doing well. Weight training with the goal of achieving a significant increase in muscular size is no exception. This concept is easy to grasp. And weight training is an easy thing to do. Granted, hitting the weights for the purpose of building a good deal of muscle can be very hard work—but other than putting forth the effort required, there just isn't much to it. It certainly doesn't seem like a discussion of the topic could fill a whole book. However, there is one problem.

Most people who attempt to build a good deal of muscle fail. Sure, almost everyone is able to gain a small amount of muscle, but many never get beyond a certain level of development, despite focused efforts, years in the gym, supplementation, adequate diet, and—not least among these—an abundance of desire. There are reasons for the widespread failure, the most common being the plain, simple, and unfortunate fact that the majority of weight trainers don't know what they're doing. The exceedingly rudimentary nature of the undertaking suggests that an equally simple approach will suffice: *Just lift weights* many think to themselves as they hit the gym and unleash a furious, nonsensical workout. *Just lift weights and good things will happen. The muscles will grow. Work a little harder and they'll grow a little more.* The idea is intuitive and simple. The act couldn't be simpler. Many think this way, and many fail. Most think they know what they're doing.

Most have some reason to believe that they do. In the beginning, results come quickly. For the beginner, almost no matter how the body is trained, an increase in muscle mass is a near certainty. This effect has positive and very often negative consequences. The benefit is that part of the goal has been accomplished: There has been a noticeable increase in muscle mass. The increase doesn't amount to much, but building a lot of muscle takes a very long time. Nevertheless, the process has begun, and some of the building has taken place.

The negative consequence of the early, initial gain is easy to fathom once it is considered that human behavior is often merely response to reinforcement: The initial gain of muscle mass reinforced the behavior that caused it. This behavior was the act of lifting weights, of using a strategy of training that might have been good, bad, or somewhere in between. The initial weeks or months of weight training are almost invariably with a bad strategy, as many approach the task with little or no direction, and probably an equal number with bad direction.

The initial gains in mass have come nonetheless. The weight trainer has been rewarded. Predictably, the beginner associates the rewards with the activity, the gains with the training. Satisfied with his initial progress, he continues along the same path. Then things begin to change. Progress often slows and then might even stop within a short period of time, typically a couple of months, a little more for some. But the training continues. The sixth-century Zen Master Bodhidharma once observed that "all know the way, but few actually walk it."[1] When considering the majority of new weight trainers, a nearly opposite observation might fit well: Many walk the path, but few know the way.

The reinforcement of muscle growth has now become randomized, because the behavior has stopped consistently generating the reinforcement. For the most part, the workouts no longer work. Humans respond to reinforcement, but they respond to random reinforcement as well, often with greater vigor. Since the training did at one time produce favorable results, it is assumed to be mainly correct. Occasionally for various reasons the growth might resume, at least for a short while, and the reinforcement is therefore truly randomized: *Sometimes the training works, so keep doing it.* The new weight trainer is left to assume—or he is assured by others—that the declining or intermittent progress is normal.

Apart from occasional, random, and typically slight increases in size, the training strategy often then produces a new kind of reward, that of allowing the weight trainer to maintain whatever gains he was able to generate. The reinforcement of maintenance, though far less compelling or exciting than the reward of growth, is often good enough to mandate a continuation of the effort. Part of the motivation to continue is often born of a fear of losing size. This association leads to further and more specifically destructive consequences.

Like all living organisms, humans are destructible. Weight training can increase size, strength, and sometimes even happiness. But weight training can be hard on the body, and can even destroy parts of it. A weight training regiment fueled by fear of losing size often becomes excessive in frequency; many will resist interspersing training with rest due to this fear, even though rest is necessary. Many simply aren't fully aware of the importance of rest and recovery. The direct consequences are twofold: Insufficient recovery will impede progress, and it will invite injury. The latter constitutes destruction of the body, the former the destruction of time.

Often and before long the reinforcement of muscle gain, now fully elusive, becomes the object of a quest. Not many settle into the complacent maintenance phase without one, or several, or even scores of attempts to break out. These forays are often comprised of further excess: More exercises, more sets, fewer days off. Workout routines are changed. The new routines are rarely improvements on the old, but it's typical at first to think that the new routine will always be better, just because it's new. For many, it is a tiresome, never-ending cycle. Sometimes this goes on for years, and a multitude has shared the experience. The brass ring just cannot be reached.

There must be a reason.

One thing everyone seems to be aware of is that there is a genetic limitation for how much muscle mass any one individual is capable of gaining. This is true—and with all weight trainers considered together, a range of limitation exists. Some people are simply able to gain more muscle than others. Only a select few can attain a degree of muscle mass of the first order, but the first order of anything is by definition reserved for a small minority. Nevertheless, everyone has the ability to significantly increase his size. But when the results of weight training are consistently disappointing, many are forced to conclude that they are the owners of bad genes. Thus, disappointing results have been identified as the problem itself; the weight trainer was doomed to fail from the very beginning, due to the irreversible blunder of having chosen the wrong parents. But a disappointing result is an outcome; it is not a problem.

The problem is a lack of knowledge.

In the life of a young child, a rather important milestone is reached when he is first able to ask the question "why?" In one sense, the ability to so inquire sets humans apart from other life forms. The child has therefore—at least in this one respect—joined humanity, the intellectual species. It also represents a developmental turning point for that particular child, since he has come to grasp the concept of causation. Delighted at their son's inquisitiveness, the happy parents answer his question. Another "why" question is asked, and another answer follows. This happens over and over, the patient parents answering away. The process continues for some time, then eventually slows down, then fades away. Apparently, by the time many of these people decide to join a gym and undertake a campaign of weight training, the word had been forgotten altogether.

Most will employ a training strategy without even considering to ask why it should be effective. They merely assume that it will be. And if they never asked in the first place, certainly they would not be able to articulate why their plan should be effective now. With this considered, it is little wonder that so many are dissatisfied with their results. Huddling within the "bad genes" cave isn't bringing them any closer to the light, either.

This book is for those who ask why.

For those who elect to inquire of the science of bodybuilding, who choose to step into the light, this is will be an exploration quite distinct from the plight of the masses described above. Just be prepared to forget everything you think you might know about weight training, because it might all be wrong! As the above must suggest, bodybuilding often takes more than just lifting weights. The first objective when beginning any undertaking should be to determine what is required in order to succeed. Success in weight training *should* include an understanding of its theoretical foundation, a determination of how that theory can be applied in the actual training sessions, and a perception of how the application can be fully optimized. Though not an absolute requisite, knowledge and understanding can only increase the odds of success. A thorough understanding of the complete process of a successful weight training campaign does require knowledge of the three aforementioned elements:

1. Theory. Lifting weights can cause muscles to grow, but sometimes lifting weights does not accomplish this. For a training strategy to insure success, it cannot be based on a randomly or arbitrarily constructed system; it must reflect a viable theory for muscular growth.
2. Execution. There are a large variety of training tactics and exercises available: Some are effective, some not. A detailed examination of the soundness and effectiveness of each is secondary only to theory in importance. The tactics and exercises of a successful effort should seek to efficiently apply the theory's assertions.
3. Intangible factors. These concern various issues of motivation but are rarely considered in detail. Intangible factors drive the entire effort, and a weight training campaign simply cannot exist without their presence—and cannot excel without their exploitation.

Knowledge is good—the more the better. The act of building muscle by lifting weights is a scientific process. All serious weight trainers have a vested interest in understanding that process. Nevertheless, most will choose a workout routine because it was something recommended by a friend, read in a magazine, or crafted individually. A few enjoy a good deal of success by doing this. They show up at the gym and crank out training sessions that give good results. They don't worry about the process causing the effect. As far as they are concerned, lifting weights causes muscles to grow, period. It is true that lifting weights can cause muscles to grow, but there are other factors in the complete cause and effect equation. If these other factors did not exist, then all weightlifting strategies would give satisfying results—which they don't. The purpose of this book is to provide the knowledge that can lead to an effective, efficient, safe, and satisfying campaign in weight training. Although it can be very hard work, weight training is an easy thing to do. But for it to be successful, it requires a good plan.

II

Intellect

"Intellect without will is worthless. Will without intellect is dangerous."

-Hans Von Seeckt

Strategy

The single most critical factor for any weight training campaign is its overall strategy. Everyone that trains with weights has an overall strategy, whether he knows and can describe it or not. Most strategies appear to be de facto in nature, because most weight trainers begin by paying close attention to determining particulars, such as certain exercises, number of sets and reps, which days ought to be spent in the gym, and countless other variables. For these people, their strategy instead becomes merely a summary of the particulars. When preparing for the invasion of Normandy, General Eisenhower did not ask his lieutenants to plan their own objectives so that he could compile the proposals, piece them all together, and then deduce what the overall attack would look like. Quite naturally, the opposite occurred: Eisenhower created the grand strategy. The subsequent planning of his subordinates all had a singular purpose— to insure the success of that plan.

The same should be true with weight training. Identifying a strategy is critical. Since no universal weight training strategy exists, there is no shortage of disagreement regarding which is best. Discounting a number of lesser variations, for quite some time there have been two primary, diametrically opposite strategies:

1. High-volume training (known also as simply "volume training"), which emphasizes a large number of sets per workout, and includes a good deal of flexibility concerning its other attributes. High-volume training was employed most notably by Arnold Schwarzenegger.
2. Low-volume, high-intensity training (HIT), which specifies that workouts should be brief, intense, and infrequent. This approach originated from the theories of Arthur Jones and the idea was refined by the late former professional bodybuilder Mike Mentzer. The idea's most visible proponent was six-time Mr. Olympia Dorian Yates.

Volume training, part one

Volume training is the strategy employed by a large majority of weight trainers. It is in fact so commonplace that in most circumstances the word "volume" is removed when speaking of it. The prominent feature of this approach is flexibility: Volume training workouts include wide ranges of sets and exercises, rep schemes, recovery times, and an almost unlimited number of weight training tactics. The strategy asserts that it can be detrimental to perform an inadequate number of sets for any exercise, and that for optimum results a high or sometimes very high number of sets—a large volume of work—should be employed.

Volume trainers strive to follow or devise training regiments possessing an ideal combination of sets, reps, exercises, and recovery periods. These routines are constructed in an attempt to reflect a particular individual's unique demands and experience level. Beginners are typically instructed to perform three sets per exercise, with perhaps three or four exercises per body part. As time passes, it is common to include more sets and exercises, the belief being that the body had become accustomed to the demands of the old regiment. Weight training routines in magazines often describe a far greater volume of work—sometimes as many as 20, 30 or even 40 sets per single body part—along with a caution that such routines are only for experts, who after many years of brutal effort have produced the ability to withstand such workouts and reap their rewards. When compared to other physical pursuits, this advice appears sensible.

Anyone deciding to enter the Los Angeles marathon yet who has never run more than a mile since high school physical education class would be ill-advised to so attempt. Such a race may be a possibility in the distant future for this person, but he must endure a great amount of strenuous and ever-lengthening training first. The idea of the progression of volume with weight training is similar. Many will gradually work their way up to longer and longer sessions. And like the runner who eventually reaches his distance goal, the progression of volume is not infinite. In an ideal scenario, the weight trainer will come to realize the appropriate threshold of volume, and he will have found what he believes to be the perfect regiment. But unlike the 26.2 miles of a marathon, the ultimate level of volume in training is flexible and dependent upon the individual.

Volume training is predicated on the idea that the act of lifting weights will cause muscles to grow. Each set in a workout will cause a little more growth than the last, so for dramatic growth it is advisable—time permitting—to perform rather extensive workouts. Since energy levels are finite, some volume sessions are concluded when the weight trainer is too exhausted to continue. To remedy this, some opt for multiple daily gym visits. Apart from economizing overall energy levels, multiple gym visits ensure that certain body parts can be trained harder than normal. A very long single workout might feature as many as four body parts. Since energy levels diminish as time passes, it's easy to imagine that the last few exercises in the session will suffer from lower energy levels. Splitting the workout into two parts with several hours of rest in between will reduce this problem. The volume strategy asserts that to get good results, a good deal of effort must go into every set.

Recovery time is considered to be important. There is a fairly wide range of recovery periods employed by volume trainers. Some train each body part as often as three times a week, some just once. The vast majority seem to fall somewhere in the middle. The idea is that this rest period will allow the muscles to rest and grow, and each subject is left to decide what amount of time is ideal for him.

Finally, volume training requires progression. The progression of volume was mentioned above. Additionally, to grow larger, the amount of weight being used must increase periodically. The volume training strategy therefore implies that an ideal scenario would include using progressively heavier weights in progressively longer workouts—until the ideal training volume has been determined.

Volume training has enjoyed massive popularity because it is straightforward, easy-to-understand, and intuitive. It has also been used by a large number of champion bodybuilders, which proves that it can work. The flexibility of the volume training idea is in every way a product of the fact that it has few, if any, hard-and-fast rules. This is little wonder, because the volume training idea emerged from unknown origins. No one knows who first came up with the idea, yet it has been in use since the dawn of weightlifting equipment, probably long before that. And this might be the single greatest reason for its popularity: It is tradition.

High-intensity training

High-intensity training is quite different from the volume variety, both in origins and execution. It was devised to be a practical application of a scientific theory regarding the human body's adaptation to stress. It also directly opposes the volume training idea that the amount of muscular growth one experiences is proportional to the number of sets used in a workout. HIT theory asserts that muscular growth is stimulated by executing training sessions of the highest possible intensity. Insofar as it is possible to produce maximum effort for only a very short duration, and owing to the HIT assertion that it is counterproductive to continue training once stimulation has been achieved, each workout should be brief. Each workout should in fact be so brief that after warming up, no more than a single working set per exercise should be employed. A complete session might include a few exercises per body part, and perhaps two or three body parts per session. A suitable degree of stimulation having been achieved for each targeted muscle group, the subject should then conclude the session. Finally, high-intensity theory mandates that a suitable amount of time must pass before the next training session, so that the body has been given adequate time to repair itself and grow—hence the "brief, intense, and infrequent" maxim of the strategy.

Volume training has enjoyed great popularity, and the opposite is true for high-intensity training, for three reasons:

1. HIT is anti-traditional, and a rebuke of tradition is often met with apprehension or even the ire of the mob.
2. It is counterintuitive. With nearly everything in life, putting in extra hours will yield greater returns; HIT asserts the opposite, that less is more. Many refuse to believe short workouts can be effective, and they do not find compelling the idea that simple stimulation is sufficient to cause growth.
3. There exists the undeniable truth that volume training is capable of producing excellent results: Many top bodybuilders' physiques are the result of volume training. Many have therefore reasoned that it can be the only effective strategy for muscle growth.

Mentzer had a few amusing responses to high-intensity training objections. Speaking to a doubter of the idea that simple simulation leads to muscular growth, he pointed out that it only takes a single sperm cell to stimulate an egg to create an entire human being.[2] Regarding the proof that many top bodybuilders' physiques are the result of volume training, he replied "so are the physiques of all the failures, whose numbers are legion."[3] Concerning the first point, it should almost go without saying that humans, though intellectually progressive, naturally cling to tradition; human history documents countless struggles to separate the two.

Despite its lower popularity, two things have helped perpetuate high-intensity training. It is as effective as the traditional volume method, and arguably more so. It has worked exceedingly well for Dorian Yates, the former professional bodybuilders Mike Mentzer, Aaron Baker, and Casey Viator—as well as myself, and a large number of successful weight trainers who nevertheless remain unknown due to a lack of desire to enter bodybuilding contests. The second point, and one that makes this strategy truly unique, is that it has a theoretical foundation. As unexpected as it may seem, within the relatively obscure microcosm of weight training for mass we find the classic confrontation of tradition versus science.

The scientific cornerstone of high-intensity training theory is a physiological mechanism called the "general adaptation syndrome" that was first postulated by the endocrinologist Hans Selye.[4] According to Selye, when an organism encounters stress, its body adapts so that it may deal with further, similar stress more effectively—and be better protected from it. The critical assertion of his theory—the assertion from which all high-intensity weight training derives—is that the degree of the body's response is proportional to the intensity of the stress it encounters.

The Adaptation Principle

Exercise is a form of stress. The body will adapt to the stress of exercise so that the next time it is encountered it will have reduced impact; it will be less stressful. In the case of endurance athletes, the body will adjust to stressful cardiovascular demands by increasing its cardiovascular capacity. But when considering the physiques of athletes such as long distance runners, it is easy to come to the conclusion that endurance sports are not an effective means to build muscle. Indeed, although the cardiovascular demands of distance running are great, the runners' muscles are subject to only very low-intensity contractions. Since the stress of these contractions is very frequent and repetitive but of minimal intensity, the body need not respond with adaptation that is more than minimal—so the result is not a significant, or even noticeable, increase in muscle mass.

Sprinters are also runners, but they have significantly different physiques than long-distance-types, with much more muscular legs. The distances they run are much shorter, and the contractions their leg muscles produce are far more intense. The same goes for speed skaters. Their bodies have responded to the short bouts of concentrated exercise— the stress of intense muscular contractions—by adapting accordingly and building larger, more powerful muscles. As can clearly be seen, the degree of the body's response rises with the intensity of the stress. Even more intense and therefore more stressful exercise produces an even greater adaptation by the body in the case of weightlifters and bodybuilders. The stress of lifting very heavy weights to and beyond failure has created the largest muscles the world has ever known.

But the development of the body's adaptive response mechanism did not come about as an anticipation of athletic competition and certainly not aesthetic improvement. Indeed, as a general adaptation mechanism, its effects can be seen in a variety of responses to stress. Probably the most commonly-cited is the body's response to direct exposure to sunlight. During the winter an entire day can be spent in the sun without a shirt or any type of sunblock, without getting a tan, and certainly not a sunburn (let's say it's a typical northern California January day, sunny and 56 degrees Farenheit). In contrast, a mere hour in Death Valley in July (115 degrees) with no shirt or sunblock will produce a significantly different response: A sunburn and eventually a tan will result, due to the greatly elevated intensity of the stress.

In the former example, since the intensity of stress was very low, the degree of the body's response would be minimal or nil. In the latter, the body reacted by causing the skin to tan so that it would be better prepared to deal with the stress of that type and degree, should the stress present itself again. An intermediate example would cause intermediate results. Observation and experimentation have shown that skeletal muscles exhibit a stress-response mechanism that is entirely consistent with the general adaptation syndrome, and it's easy to see how intense radiation creating a tan is analogous to intense muscular contractions resulting in muscular growth.

The body's mechanism for adaptation is actually the sixth principle of high-intensity theory, originally outlined by Mentzer. It has been mentioned here first because it directly addresses the question of why muscles grow. But before discussing the remaining principles, it is worth mentioning what is meant by *theory*, since it is in this most general sense that high-intensity is differentiated from many other types of training. Webster's Dictionary offers the following definition: It is "a plausible or scientifically acceptable general principle or body of principles offered to explain phenomena." Additionally, any viable theory should be able to predict future occurrences and can be confirmed or falsified through experiment or observation. High-intensity training is an instance of a scientifically acceptable idea, or conclusion, arrived at by combining a set of scientifically acceptable principles. Its predicted effects have been confirmed through observation. The body's ability to adapt is one of its principles.

The Identity Principle

The Identity Principle states that we have a physiological identity, in that we are all human beings. While all humans have a unique genetic makeup, with corresponding differences in muscle shape, length, and density, height, eye, hair, and skin color, predisposition to body fat storage, and countless other attributes, we all share a common physiology. Our organs all function in the same way, and we all possess the same physiological mechanisms, one such being the general adaptation syndrome. Inasmuch, there can be only one correct scientific explanation for the cause-and-effect relationship of exercise and muscle mass building for all human beings.

It is common for bodybuilders to advocate an experimental approach to weight training, since an equally common misconception is that "everyone is different." While it might be true that an exercise might be more effective for one person than for another due to, for instance, subtle mechanical discrepancies between the two—an example being bench press, which works wonderfully for some people but not so much for others—the two subjects still share the same physiology, and will build muscle due to the same physiological processes. However, the advocacy of experimentation often extends to the construction of fundamentally disparate training strategies, the implication being that we have different physiologies to an equally fundamental degree. This is incorrect. If it were to be so, there would be no medical profession as we now know it, since it would be far too difficult to keep track of all the different physiologies possessed by humans. Thankfully this is not the case, and in a general physiological sense it can be said with certainty that we are all the same.

The Intensity Principle

The above discussion of the Adaptation Principle made several references to the idea that the degree of the body's response is proportional to the intensity of stress it encounters. It is therefore necessary, if one wishes to elicit the most dramatic muscular growth, to subject his muscles to the most intense contractions possible. There are a few weight-training tactics that can be used in order to achieve such stimulation, and these will be addressed in the *Physique* section. Meanwhile, once again consider the examples of adaptation with regard to runners, sprinters, and weightlifters. As the intensity of contractions associated with these activities rise, so do the degrees of the body's adaptive response: The greater the intensity, the greater the growth. Physiological research has shown that intensity is the only important exercise factor in muscular growth.[5]

Intensity is a relative term. "Maximum" intensity refers to highest possible momentary muscular effort. "High" intensity refers to the highest level of momentary muscular effort the subject can muster. This is not maximum, but close to it. Maximum intensity should be the desired level in any workout whose purpose is to build muscle mass. However, human energy levels are finite. A workout cannot go on for very long if the subject requires that maximum or very high levels of intensity occur with each set. In a weightlifting workout, with each successive set, the level of intensity—relative to the level possible had the subject approached it "fresh"—will drop: The longer the workout, the further the drop. Although a subject might be trying his hardest, the level of intensity of any set he performs late in a volume-oriented workout will not be close to maximum, so it cannot be considered high.

The actual level of intensity of these sets will vary from individual to individual. Some unfortunate weight trainers seem unable to generate high levels of intensity, even on the first working set. There are also the rare anomalies, famous for accomplishing brutal workouts, who seem to be able to generate high levels of intensity through extensive workouts. As will be seen, this can turn out to be a rather destructive combination, often resulting in even greater misfortune. In general, however, maximum intensity cannot be maintained for more than very brief periods.

Since the aim of an effective mass-building workout should be to produce highest possible level of intensity of muscular contractions, it helps to be aware of the fact that there are three types of muscular strength: Concentric, static, and eccentric. In simple terms, the concentric portion of an exercise is the lifting, or positive segment; the static portion involves holding the weight motionless at any point in the range of movement of the exercise; and the eccentric, or negative portion, involves lowering of the weight (under control, not dropping the weight while hanging on to it).

Sets are often performed in a manner such that the subject reaches failure in only the concentric portion of the movement. It is common to see people in gyms training until positive failure, and then terminating the set. This is particularly true with bench presses; typically the subject will perform as many reps as possible. Once positive failure has been reached, he will get assistance from his spotter on subsequent reps. However, rather than lowering the weight in a slow, controlled fashion, which will help him reach failure in the negative portion of the movement, the subject more or less drops the weight to the bottom position, often with the aid by the spotter, and uses the "bounce" to help him perform the next rep.

Since it is in the concentric portion of any movement where muscles are at their weakest, this is where they will always first fail—and the mistake is often made that positive failure should signal the end of a set. Training to positive failure is a good idea early in a weight training campaign, but later on—maybe a few months down the road—more intense contractions become necessary. When training to positive failure, maximum-intensity contractions have not yet taken place. Muscles are strongest during the eccentric phase, and this fact must be exploited in order to achieve maximum-intensity contractions.

An ideal bench-pressing scenario would include the following amendment to the last example: After reaching positive failure, instead of dropping the weight to the bottom position, the subject should lower the weight in a very slow, controlled, and unassisted manner to the bottom position. If at this point negative failure has not been reached, and the subject feels that he is able to complete another repetition where the weight is brought down slowly and deliberately, then he should do so. The set should be continued until the subject cannot lower the weight with control. At this point failure truly has been reached, and muscle should have been sufficiently stimulated. The example of this particular technique is intended for advanced lifters, and additional details will be given in the *Physique* section.

Obviously stimulation with this degree of intensity is not achieved by the sprinter, and the difference in results between the leg sizes of bodybuilders and sprinters is ample testimony to this. The distance runner's contractions are an even further remote comparison, and contrasting the thigh measurements of bodybuilders and marathoners mirrors this dissimilarity.

In order to successfully embark on a high-intensity training regiment, one must master the ability to generate, on demand, physical effort of the highest order. Since the degree of the body's response rises in proportion to the intensity of the stress it experiences, the importance of achieving highly intense workouts should not be underestimated.

The Duration Principle

Since it has been established that for the purposes of maximum stimulation and growth, intensity of muscular contractions should be of the highest order, it logically follows that training sessions should be, and in fact *must be* brief. Very high-intensity output can be maintained for only a very short period of time; the longer a training session drags on, the less intense it will become. Consider again the long-distance runner. The muscular contractions he is able to perform can only be of very low intensity, otherwise he would tire too quickly and never finish the race. A sprinter, running much faster, is generating far more intense contractions—but imagine if he tried to run a marathon while maintaining the speed and intensity of a 100-meter dash. He wouldn't get far.

A workout cannot both be long and intense. Since an optimal muscle-building training session must be as intense as possible, it therefore must be brief. It is possible to start a training session with an all-out effort, but any attempt to maintain this intensity as the workout wears on will fail. But let's suppose that intense output can be maintained indefinitely. In this case, it would still make sense to make the training session brief; any sets performed for a particular exercise beyond a single high-intensity set would be meaningless, because there is no benefit to be gained from another set of equal intensity. The stimulation from intense muscular contractions is not cumulative.

But in the real world, where our energy reserves are finite, subsequent sets are more and more likely to be of lesser intensity as the workout continues. As the training drags on, they *must* become less intense. And since the body responds in kind to the intensity of stress it receives, what good is it to perform lower-intensity sets? Other than burning a few extra calories, such sets certainly serve no purpose, and are actually rather harmful. The body must devote more resources to repairing the acute damage caused by the additional training. The muscles have been excessively broken down, but by performing unnecessary sets the subject also inches ever closer to joint damage, something countless volume trainers have found to be inevitable. Additionally, excessive training taxes the body in a general sense.

I recall in my days as a volume trainer many years ago that I would conclude each workout as if I were limping across the finish line of a long race. I had given my muscles a thorough pounding, and I thought that this hard work—that I have long-since realized was badly misplaced—would be the key to my success. There was a period when I was training shoulders, biceps, and triceps all in a single session. Looking back, I was probably performing as many as 50 total sets on that day, *not* including warm-ups! My last few sets were downright loathsome.

I was spent, completely drained, and I couldn't wait for the workout to be over. As one might imagine, by the end the intensity I was able to generate was poor. I did *try*; I would reach down deep into my psyche in an attempt to scrape up as much motivation as possible—but no matter how much drive an individual has, his energy reserves are limited. I was performing high-intensity sets beyond failure, but I was also performing a great deal of redundant, superfluous, and counterproductive work as well. I was obviously not keeping each workout brief.

Eventually my training changed. Although I had come to accept the idea that more is *not* better, I will admit that once I embarked upon a high-intensity training regiment, I would often conclude a workout with some lingering apprehension. I was used to long, grueling hours in the gym, along with a feeling upon leaving the gym of exhaustion. After completing an effective high-intensity workout, one should not be exhausted.

High-intensity training will *not* drain you, and you should *not* feel as if you can't wait for a HIT workout to end. So at first, this was the source of my apprehension: With volume training, I was used to being completely worn-out afterwards. And since I had at least a little success with this strategy, I did associate this success with the drained feeling. And, to be honest, even to someone who understands the logic completely, it's hard to fully reject the "more is better" impulse, even if it only exists on a subconscious level. But one must believe in his own conscious intellect, just as he will do himself an injustice by basing his decisions on tradition or even superstition rather than logic.

It might help to once more consider that mammals respond to random reinforcement. A rat will push a lever down if a pellet of food is dispensed as a result. Each time the lever is pushed, another pellet is released. In a famous psychological experiment, the rat in question later began to receive a pellet after pushing the bar twice, then ten times, then every one hundred times. Rats have been observed to press the lever more than a thousand times, all because once in a while the behavior of pressing the lever is rewarded. Such is the case with excessively long workouts. Often times, particularly very early on in a weight training campaign, *any* type of workout will produce results. The reinforcement has thus begun. Even if the subject's progress slows or stops altogether, or even if it occasionally resumes (which will normally take place after a sizable layoff), the original reinforcement is there—and the inefficient and exhausting workouts continue in the hopes of receiving the elusive rewards.

High-intensity training is very difficult physically and requires a completely different mastery of the mental/motivational angle than volume training, since one must have the ability to create a mental state which will allow for absolute maximum effort when it is needed. But high-intensity training is not difficult in the sense that a 50-set volume workout is difficult—nor is it hard the way finishing a marathon or climbing a 20,000 foot mountain peak is hard. In volume training, one must have the head-down, *keep going* attitude of the long distance runner or mountain climber. With high-intensity training, one must have the ability to unleash a torrent of effort at the precise moment it is required, and he must be prepared to accept the fact that he will not be exhausted at the end of a training session which, to be optimally effective, must be brief.

The Frequency Principle

Whereas training sessions are meant to stimulate growth, the actual growth occurs during periods of rest. It is therefore necessary to allow for an adequate amount of time to elapse between training sessions. After the problem of excessive volume, the second most common mistake made by bodybuilders and weightlifters concerns the issue of frequency: Most lifters will train too often. This problem is compounded by the fact that most gym-goers will perform a high volume of work as well, which apart from being by itself counterproductive, requires an even greater period of rest. Combining the two biggest mistakes in bodybuilding is a sure path to failure.

Training with weights breaks down muscle tissue, and a certain amount of time must elapse before the tissue is able to restore itself. Assuming that the training session in question was adequate to stimulate muscular growth, a subsequent period must elapse for this growth to take place. The amount of time that must pass for the first phase to be completed varies from subject to subject. Some studies have demonstrated that this initial repair can occur in as little as 36 hours, while others suggest that the period for recovery could be significantly longer.

Apart from that, intense weight training taxes the body in a general sense, and some research has suggested that the central nervous system requires a greater recovery period than the muscles themselves when the high-intensity variety is employed.[6] Whether or not that is truly the case, it has been well-documented that an overtrained state can be induced by exercise of low intensity and high duration, such as long-distance running, or by medium-intensity, medium-duration ventures such as volume weight-training. So even if the muscles themselves are not heavily broken down, it is still possible to run one's self ragged by employing a routine of high volume and frequency. Routines employing a "double-split," where the subject will visit the gym twice in a day, will nudge the subject even closer to (or plunge him deeper into) such a state.

Since it is impossible for the average subject to observe, under laboratory conditions, the repair as it transpires, it then falls upon him to form a subjective albeit educated estimate of his own recovery requirements. Since the mid-1980s, the recommended rest period that should take place between any two workouts for the same body part has been increasing. There is an undeniable correlation between the increased rest and increased mass among top bodybuilders during this period, and although there are certainly other factors in the equation, evidently the extra rest has helped.

Of course it is natural to assume that the greatest worry to arise from employing an extended-rest strategy would be that the subject would be *under*training—which, although a legitimate concern, is a problem bordering on nonexistence. Almost no one throws in the towel due to a lack of progress induced by not training enough. The drive that propels one to visit the gym regularly for years tends to spill over into over-enthusiasm, which when left unabated will almost always cause the subject to train too much and too often. Since (and rather incredibly) few approach the idea of formulating a sensible training strategy with much more than casual interest, the numbers that even consider the possibility that they might be inviting overtraining due to excessive workout frequency are slim. Those who do not possess a great deal of enthusiasm for training, who are theoretically more likely candidates for undertraining, tend to take extended breaks from it which can last for months or even years. This isn't really "undertraining," as it seems to be more a case of intermittent-training or non-training.

So the primary concern is that one should not train too frequently. Selecting a proper frequency of workouts insures that adequate time has been devoted to repair and growth—and it also insures that overtraining will be avoided. An overtrained state will cause all progress to cease, and often times the subject will become weaker, smaller, and softer—exactly the opposite of what he had hoped to achieve.

The obvious question then becomes "how much rest is ideal?" As this will vary from subject to subject, no single answer is correct. Beginners are fine with a relatively high frequency, training each body part two or even three times per week, as the aim should be acclimation rather than maximum intensity. Once he begins, in earnest, a high-intensity program, allowing four days of rest before training any single body part again should be considered minimum. It should then be left to the subject to determine, as time passes, if this is enough rest. This isn't necessarily an easy task for a beginner.

The most obvious indicator will be the subject's progress. One should ask himself "am I stronger?" and "am I bigger?" With this in mind, he should keep close track of his progression. Granted, there can be quite few variables to consider, such as diet, intensity of effort, supplements, etc, but during the first year or so of training, gains in strength and mass should be steady and noticeable. If progress is slow or has stopped, excessive frequency might be the culprit. Another less objective method to assess frequency is to appraise one's own motivation. It should be easy to get motivated to train. If the subject should find himself not looking forward to or even dreading the gym, that sentiment should be taken seriously. Disintegrating enthusiasm tends to be a very reliable sign that one's efforts are excessive—whether the excess occurs in volume or frequency or both.

As the subject becomes more massive, he must generate ever-increasing intensity levels during his training sessions to grow even further, and the length of time for adequate recovery will increase as well. Over the years I endured such an evolution, and for many of those years I enjoyed excellent results training each body part once a week. Such a regiment is now fairly common practice among bodybuilders, an uncharacteristically sensible transition from the twice-a-week dogma that was dominant little more than 20 years ago. Around that time it was considered fairly radical for a bodybuilder to switch to the new three-on, one-off strategy; world champion Lee Haney adopted it, and it thus became the new vogue. A few years later came the four-on, one-off idea, considered equally radical. Eventually weekly training took hold, although large numbers still train more frequently. As for me, I will often feel an overtrained state coming on if I train any single body part more than once every eight days.

There is no clear-cut answer to the question of how often one must train to get optimal results. That is for each individual to decide, much as one must decide which combination of exercises will suit him best. The important point is regardless of the number of days that should elapse, it is critical that enough time passes so that one may allow his body to recover and grow.

The Specificity Principle

The idea here is that specific forms of exercise are required to achieve specific results. Once more the examples of long-distance runners, sprinters, and bodybuilders can be considered. The distance runner's goal is to achieve the highest level possible of cardiovascular and muscular endurance, so that he might run farther—or in the case of training to run a pre-set distance such as a marathon, that he might do so more quickly. To effectively reach these goals, a specific form of training should be employed.

The sprinter is also concerned with running a certain distance for a faster time than what his previous efforts had produced, although obviously the specific training he will employ will be quite a bit different than the distance runner, since he is concerned with covering 100 meters as quickly as possible rather than 26 miles. If on the day of the track meet the sprinter and the distance runner are instructed to switch places, so that each will be running in the other's race, both should be expected to fail miserably, since their training was specific to the wrong event.

The bodybuilder, whose aim should be to build as much mass as possible, also needs to employ methods of training that are specific to that goal. There is one difference, however: To excel at running, the runner runs; to excel at sprinting, the sprinter sprints; but to add muscle mass, the bodybuilder trains for *strength*. The mass he will add is a by-product of that effort. All things being equal, a muscle that is made stronger will be made bigger. There are no known instances of someone increasing his muscle mass without getting stronger.

Apart from selecting a form of training that is specifically designed to produce greater strength and therefore mass, the subject ought to specifically avoid training that will detract from this effort. It has already been pointed out that the two most common errors committed by bodybuilders are excessive volume and frequency, and obviously these should be avoided.

Apart from problems with the strategy itself, many volume-trainers adhere to misplaced specificity, thinking that certain forms of training are required to achieve a particular "look." A commonly-held belief is that, particularly before bodybuilding contests, there ought to be a relatively quick pace to a workout. From a practical standpoint, the increased pace helps to accommodate the increased volume of workload—in the form of additional exercises, sets, and reps—that the subject will impose upon himself as the contest nears. The reasoning here is that the fast pace and extra volume will somehow improve his appearance.

The reasoning here is unclear. Is the fast pace supposed to raise one's heart rate over a certain level for a long enough period of time to elicit a fat-burning effect? This is certainly possible. However:

1. The intensity level that one is able to devote to any particular set will suffer markedly.
2. The number of sets that must be performed in order to keep one's heart rate in the fat-burning range for an appreciable period of time will be staggering, and far beyond what would be optimal for stimulating muscular growth.
3. The large number of total sets will very likely cause an overtrained state, despite the impaired intensity level.
4. An infinitely more efficient and effective method specifies a clear division of weight and cardio work.

The problem is that those that will perform the light, fast, and lengthy weight workouts for the most part will also overdo their cardio training. Since those employing this method tend to also favor an excessively stringent dietary approach, these people tend to end up, in "contest shape," appearing flat, small, and tired. This is good news for the rational, hard-training bodybuilder that chooses to avoid this list of pitfalls.

Obviously a bodybuilder will want to reduce his body fat to minimum levels before a contest. This can be achieved through diet and cardio exercise. But the primary aim of such contests is to display large muscles, and a form of training that is specifically designed to produce maximum muscular growth should be used throughout the precontest phase. But regardless of the subject's competitive aspirations (or if he has any at all) he should always be aware of what specific training will be optimal to achieve an increase in muscle mass. The Physique section of this book addresses the specifics of weight-training for mass, both tactics and exercises.

you train with 100% intensity in one session, it is reasonable to expect that you will lift heavier weights the next time around by generating that same 100% (without having to venture into the realm of above-100% effort, which is an impossibility anyway), thus insuring another gain in mass.

There are two pitfalls regarding the idea of progression. The first is that subjects will often fail to realize the importance of it. As paradoxical as this might sound, some bodybuilders are so concerned with size that they have little concern for the amount of weight they are lifting, and they don't make an effort to at least attempt to progressively increase the weights they are using or the amount of reps they are performing.

The second problem is that many employ a progression of volume. Rather than seeking to exploit strength gains to subject their muscles to new levels of stimulation, many bodybuilders will simply add more sets to their repertoire. Once again, such a tactic is driven by the faulty "more is better" logic. Ironically, it is in the progression principle that it is truly the case that more *is* better, but in a different sense: It is still the goal to achieve optimal stimulation through a single, high-intensity set—but from one workout to the next it must be the goal to use *more weight*, or lift the same weight for *more reps*, or both. More is better!

In summary

The seven principles listed above, first outlined by Mike Mentzer[7], form a coherent theory that has been confirmed through observation and is capable of predicting future occurrences. The general idea is also easily summarized:

There is a cause-and-effect relationship between weight training and muscular growth. Human beings share a basic physiology, so this relationship applies to all people. Muscular growth occurs as a result of the stimulation of very intense exercise; as the intensity of stimulation rises, the body will adapt by increasing the amount of muscle it adds. Since a training session cannot be both intense and long, it must be brief. After sufficient muscular stimulation has been achieved, the body must be given adequate time to rest, so that it may repair itself and grow. The type of exercise used must be specifically designed for the purpose of building mass. To continue growing, the muscles must be subjected to ever-increasing levels of stress.

That's it—concise, elegant, easy-to-fathom, efficient, and effective.

Volume training, part two

It is easy to see how the volume training approach might stumble once brought into the light of skeptical analysis. The one principle that forms the foundation of various volume training strategies seems to be merely "more is better." This is a slightly puzzling assertion considering there is no accompanying attempt to describe *why* more is better, just that it is. Nor is there a rational formula for determining the ideal volume threshold, the point beyond which returns become negative. Held under scrutiny, the volume training idea becomes more suspect, its mechanism more vague, its successes more apparently anomalous.

But perhaps we should back up for a moment and give volume training a degree of examination such that we might accept or reject it based on our findings. Since the nature of science is self-correction, all theories, those regarding weight-training included, can be assessed by first examining the cogency of their principles; the theories can then be subject to repudiation, revision, or falsification through empirical observation. To not offer volume training this examination would be unfair, unscientific, and might actually subvert the plausibility of contrary opinion, at least in the eyes of casual observers. Indeed, to dismiss any idea as well as the credibility of its source without an earnest and fair investigation, no matter how illogical that idea might appear, can invigorate and even rally those who still cling to it.

One unrelated example illustrates this point well, and involves the eccentric cosmologist Emmanuel Velikovsky. In 1950 Velikovsky created a great deal of controversy in the scientific community when he boldly released *Worlds in Collision*, a book that sought to explain that phenomena in the Judeo-Christian Bible resulted from astronomical activity, or more specifically, because the Earth had near-misses with other planets of our solar system, thus setting off these events.[8] In apparent disregard for (or ignorance of) gravitational and electromagnetic effects, and indeed, physical laws in general, he offered to explain the causes, "scientifically," for a number of what were otherwise considered supernatural occurrences in the Old Testament.

His general hypothesis was presented under the name of "Catastrophism," and included, among other things, the following claims: The planet Venus, until about 1500 BC, did not occupy its current orbit; rather, it was contained inside the planet Jupiter, which then suddenly ejected it into space. At that point Venus became a comet, and had a near-collision with Earth. This near miss precipitated a number of highly unusual occurrences, not the least of which was the parting of the Red Sea. The near-miss also, due to its warming effect, stimulated the reproductive activity of frogs (causing the Egyptian frog plague). The comet was also responsible for the locust plague, manna dropping from the heavens, and number of other unlikely events. After wreaking havoc in the skies directly above the Earth, Venus then moved along, settling into what is now its present orbit. Truly, Velikovsky had made a lot of incredible claims.

Predictably, the scientific community was not impressed with Velikovsky's opus. He and his ideas were very quickly dismissed as crackpot, often times by scientists who were aware of the main points of his ideas but never actually read the book. This is understandable, considering the obvious incoherency of Catastrophism as a cosmological theory. However, to a fair number of people with strong religious convictions and lack of scientific knowledge and skepticism (or at least a willingness to ignore physical laws), Velikovsky's views were attractive. In their eyes he assumed the role of hero, and his book became a best-seller. Some compared him to ground-breaking cosmological theorists of the past, including no less than Isaac Newton and Albert Einstein. The quick and mocking dismal of the scientific community became the rallying point of his constituency; they felt he was being treated unfairly, specifically on the grounds that the scientific community had made up their minds early on that they would not accept or even entertain his ideas. Exacerbating this sentiment was the fact that Macmillan Publishers, bowing to pressure from the scientific community, agreed to stop publishing the book (the title was transferred to Doubleday).

In a sense this was something as a role reversal; much as Galileo's and Copericus's views were quickly dismissed and condemned by that period's authority on cosmological matters (the Church), Velikovsky found himself in a similar predicament with the scientific community—although of course there is a striking disparity between the specifics of the respective examples. Nevertheless, Velikovsky had unwittingly established for himself an ardent base of support, fueled by a collective feeling of exclusion and abasement.

But any idea is amenable to scientific examination, and should be afforded such, Velikovskian Catastrophism being no exception. In the spirit of this sentiment, popular scientist and educator Carl Sagan, in his book *Broca's Brain: Reflections on the Romance of Science,* addressed and analyzed a number of Velikovsky's assertions.[9] Seeking to prove through careful consideration whether any of the claims were possible, in the end he was able to dispel them all. In fact, as a scientist, it was his duty to do so. Among many of the ideas that Sagan examined was the assertion that Venus had been "ejected" from Jupiter. He produced a fairly simple calculation that demonstrated the amount of energy that would be required for such a task to have happened. As it turns out, the amount of energy required for this ejection would also create a very high temperature—a temperature so hot, in fact, that Venus would melt as a result, and its particles would be dispersed in a cloud. The event would have more closely resembled an explosion than an ejection. Therefore, the planet could not possibly have careened by the Earth, setting off Biblical plagues, and it certainly could not have then reached its ultimate destination, its current orbit, in one piece—or even in billions and billions of pieces.

Sagan applied scientific examination to several other claims, and to no surprise, these were debunked as well. I could recount the specifics, but by now the point should have been well taken. And I think I have very obviously implied the importance of giving volume training theory a fair shake. I decided that it would be best to attempt to prove or debunk, once and for all, the notion that volume training is indeed a viable theory.

After committing to pursue this effort, I immediately ran into a major problem: As far as I can tell, there is no such theory! I had been looking for a set of principles, or observations about how the human body functions and responds to stress (or more specifically, to weight training) that when considered together would prescribe a workout regiment—one similar to the volume training schemes described in magazines or on the internet, or seen perpetrated in gyms, and one that will once-and-for-all settle the issue of exactly how many sets in a volume regiment are required for optimal muscular stimulation and therefore growth. I have not been successful.

After thinking on it for a while, I realized that this was a rather astounding discovery. Countless bodybuilders and weightlifters, for several decades, have approached the problem of adding muscle mass by implementing a method that has little or no rational foundation. Not only is there no scientifically valid theory to back it up, there is no theory *at all*!

The best I could do is locate a set of bodybuilding "principles" (which are often called the "Weider Principles," purported to be the invention of renowned publishing magnate Joe Weider[10]), a few of which should look familiar to anyone who has been lifting weights or reading the magazines for any length of time. (In fact, one can observe people using any number of these on any given day, certainly far more often than high-intensity training). This compendium of ideas does not seem to collectively construct a coherent theory, nor does it appear to pretend to. Rather, at first glance it is mainly more of a somewhat disjointed collection of weight-training strategies, tactics, or at worst, nifty ideas or gimmicks by which one can supposedly trick the body into growing. But, as in the case of *Worlds in Collision*, maybe we should reserve judgment pending closer examination. The principles, in no particular order, are as follows:

Muscle Priority Training Principle

The principle

The idea here is that one should train his underdeveloped or lagging muscles first, so as to subject them to maximum possible effort. This should also insure that these muscles will be trained before fatigue sets in.

Conclusions

This principle is not incongruent per se with what we know about the body's adaptation to stress, need for recovery, or requirement of intensity of stress to elict the desired effect. However, the principle does imply that in any workout, the subject will experience a general fatigue, and that muscles not trained first will not be addressed with optimal effort. If volume training is in fact a viable theory, this is a valid concern. The principle, viewed in light of the implied length of workout (a long, volumistic affair), does not hold up well concerning what we know about the intensity of stress determining the degree of the body's response—in that it is certain that the intensity we are able to generate decreases as time passes. But maybe we can assume that lesser-intensity exercise stimulates a response in the body that is independent of, and obviously different from, the general adaptation syndrome. Such a responsive mechanism has yet to be discovered, however. Although advertised as a "principle," muscle priority training is actually more of a weight-training tactic.

Pyramiding Principle

The principle

When using multiple sets for a given exercise, the subject should perform his first set with less weight for more repetitions, gradually increasing the weight and decreasing the reps over the remainder of your sets. This allows muscles to adequately warm up, thus that they may address the subsequent, heavier weights with reduced risk of injury.

Conclusions

Warming up is an absolute necessity, especially once the subject has attained a good deal of strength. In fact, very strong muscles are far more susceptible to tearing than weak ones. The only problem I can see is that this principle does not specify which sets ought to be taken to failure or beyond, if any. If all sets are performed as warm-ups, save for the last, which the subject should take to failure or beyond, then this would be consistent with what we know about the body's adaptation to stress of exercise, resultant increases in muscular mass, and the dangers of over-training. However, since pyramiding is a scheme very frequently used in volume training, then we can assume that this is not the case, and the idea is that multiple sets are to be taken to failure or beyond. Whereas the previous principle implied the need for a bodily mechanism to reward its inclusion, this principle requires it: As mentioned previously, the idea that volume training should be considered viable requires that the body have a mechanism that allows it to count sets or reward extended-duration efforts. Again, none has been discovered. As with muscle priority training, this is a tactic, not a principle.

Set System Training Principle

The principle

Set system training prescribes that one should perform more than one set per exercise. This principle was apparently devised as a reaction to high-intensity training. The belief here is that the first set, or even the first few sets, are not adequate to fully stimulate growth—or, in the words of Fred Hatfield, Ph.D., multiple sets per exercise are advised "in order to apply maximum adaptive stress."[11]

Conclusions

Here we have it in writing: More is better. This is actually the principle that would come closest to forming the basis of a volume training theory, if one were to exist. Of course, along with this assertion, we will need an explicit description of *why* more is better. I have already discussed at some length the problems with this idea. Worthy of note is that Hatfield, despite being the president of the International Sports Sciences Association, in his statement has demonstrated a lack of understanding regarding a fundamental property of the body's adaptation mechanism: The degree of the body's response is proportional to intensity of stress, not duration.

Instinctive Training Principle

The principle

The idea here is that by following one's instincts, a training regiment can be changed or fine-tuned to achieve better results. As he progresses, the subject ought to develop a "feel" for how he should be training, and make changes accordingly; these changes can be in set/rep schemes, types of exercises, number of rest days, or whatever other variables the subject chooses. The instinctive training notion is predicated upon the idea that each individual has a unique physiology, and that tailoring a workout is therefore essential.

Conclusions

Instinct is behavior that occurs independently of environmental influences or conditioning; it is behavior we are born with. Humans have precious few instincts, and an impulse to lift weights is not among them. Dorian Yates once quipped that if one were to follow his instincts, he would be down at the pub chasing after women rather than lifting a barbell.

I'm not sure who coined the phrase "instinctive training," but I'll give him the benefit of the doubt and assume that what he really meant was that one should use *intuition*, rather than instinct, to devise or modify his training methods. Although it seems that this would be a more appropriate choice of words, this is still a dubious method for devising a training method. Intuition is defined as arriving at knowledge or conclusions independent of experience or conscious thought. There is certainly nothing wrong with intuition by itself; in fact a great number of man's intellectual feats were hatched through an initial intuitive thought. However, an idea arrived at through intuition should then be examined via rational, conscious consideration. And there is nothing wrong with tailoring a workout, an example being, after time, switching from one exercise to another for a certain body part—but this change should come about as a result of thoughtful analysis, not by consulting with some illusory "instinct." That being said, this is actually the first of two principles that could be invoked to modify the "more is better" precept.

Finally, apart from the rare anomaly, humans all have the same basic physiology. Devising a training plan that includes a greater number of sets than what a second subject would employ, because such training is more appropriate for that individual's unique physiology, is an idea based on imaginary constructs.

Supersets Principle

The principle

The idea here is that two sets, each for a different muscle group, ought to be performed in back-to-back fashion, with as little rest as possible. It is most commonly prescribed that these muscle groups ought to oppose each other, examples being biceps and triceps, or chest and back. It is further thought that such an approach will greatly "increase intensity" and that the extra muscle pump will translate into enhanced growth.

Conclusions

Rather than being a device to increase intensity, this method is likely to reduce intensity, since intensity of the highest order can be prolonged only for very short time. The second exercise, following the first with almost no rest, will most probably be of lower intensity and therefore not optimally productive; also, there is a risk that aerobic failure will occur before its anaerobic counterpart, and the subject will be too winded to generate proper intensity during the second half of the superset. Since it is typical that several supersets for the same muscle will be performed in a single workout (as this is part of a volume training regiment), then the muscle trained in the second half of the movement will be subject to increasingly reduced intensity. It is reasonable to expect an increased "pump," due to the fact that two muscles in the same region are trained in quick succession. However, there is no evidence that this will translate into enhanced growth. Again, this is a tactic, not a principle.

Tri-Sets Principle

The principle

This method is similar to supersets, the exception being that three sets are performed in quick succession, and are typically of three different exercises, and all exercises should work the same muscle. This is a method often used during a pre-contest phase of training.

Conclusions

For some body parts, I do not think that it's necessarily a bad idea to perform three different exercises, as it seems that a complete stimulation of all muscle fibers might be beyond the scope of any single exercise. Back training is an example of this. However, performing three sets in quick succession will naturally limit the intensity one is able to devote to the second and especially third portions of the tri-set. For the purpose of stimulating maximum muscular growth, this approach is contrary to what we know about the body's response being in proportion to intensity of stress it experiences. As for its usefulness in a bodybuilding pre-contest phase, when the idea is to shed as much subcutaneous body fat as possible, I suppose the notion is that such a tactic will burn more calories than a conventional approach. This issue will be addressed later, but it is far more effective to have a clear delineation between weight and cardio training. Again, this is a tactic, not a principle.

Giant Sets Principle

The principle

Giant sets are essentially the same as tri-sets, except that four or more exercises are performed in a row—again, with as little rest as possible between sets.

Conclusions

As with tri-sets, giant sets constitute an approach that is contrary to what we know about the body's response being in proportion to intensity of stress it experiences. In fact, giant sets are an aerobic (rather than anaerobic) exercise method, albeit one that places undue stress on the connective tissue of the particular muscles being trained. If weights are to be used for cardiovascular training, then a large variety of exercises for many different body parts should be used. Of course, cardiovascular training will only build a very slight amount of muscle in only otherwise untrained subjects. Yet again, this is a tactic, not a principle.

Compound Sets Principle

The principle

This idea is the same as tri-sets, except that only two exercises are performed in a row, with as little rest as possible, rather than three.

Conclusions

This principle has the same basic problems found with supersets and tri-sets. However, performing two different exercises in quick succession can be valuable if the guidelines of the pre-exhaustion tactic (see below) are followed. But an arbitrary pairing of two exercises for the same body part, by itself, is counterproductive. Again, this is a tactic, not a principle.

Staggered Sets Principle

The principle

The idea behind staggered sets is that a smaller, slower-developing body part ought to be trained in a manner that each set is interspersed with the training of a larger body part; each body part is trained in an alternating fashion. Arnold Schwarzenegger claimed to use this method to bring up his lagging calves; after performing a set for a larger muscle group, he would perform a set of calves, then repeat. In this way he was able to force himself to perform a large volume of calve training, up to 20 sets in a single session.

Conclusions

If more is indeed better, then this method makes sense. Again, this is a tactic, not a principle.

Double or Triple Split Training Principle

The principle

Split training is the practice of visiting the gym twice or even three times per day. Rather than performing a single, long workout, where several body parts are trained, the idea is that by resting for several hours between body parts, more energy can be devoted to each.

Conclusions

Assuming that volume training is a correct theory, then it does make sense that more energy can be devoted to each body part by splitting up a workout—since volume-oriented workouts are by definition lengthy and therefore taxing. Since our examination of the aforementioned principles has not come close to proving this assumption, then we are forced to reserve judgment pending the outcome of our findings. If it turns out that we are not able to prove that volume training is a coherent theory, then split training is completely unnecessary. Beyond that, if volume training is found to be lacking in cogency, then split training is certainly counterproductive, as visiting the gym repeatedly can lead to mental and/or physical burnout. Again, this is a tactic, not a principle.

Holistic Training Principle

The principle

The assertion here is that there are variations among the types of cellular organelles located within our muscles, and that each responds to stress uniquely. Furthermore, different set and rep schemes will cause a type of stress unique to that method. Therefore, bodybuilders should experiment with different set and rep schemes in order to figure out which combination thereof will best match the response mechanism of each organelle, thus resulting in the best possible gain in muscle mass.

Conclusions

All evidence suggests that all muscles respond in the same fashion to the stress of intense muscular contraction. Also, there are not different types of stress with regard to muscular contraction, only different degrees. Maybe this should be called the "Experimentation Principle," since the mention of cellular organelles is superfluous, and the principle is ultimately just a prescription for experimentation. There is nothing wrong with experimentation, but as muscular gains tend to come very slowly, it would be exceedingly difficult to control all the variables throughout the course of the experiment. Experimentation without theoretical underpinnings is rather unscientific, and one could spend a lifetime conducting such experiments to little avail. This is the second principle that might be used to modify the "more is better" Set System Training idea.

Eclectic Training Principle

The principle

The subject ought to combine strength, mass, and refinement training techniques, as dictated by instinct, in order to optimize muscular gains.

Conclusions

This seems to be a combination of the Instinctive and Holistic training principles. It would be tempting to dismiss this idea in the spirit of "two wrongs don't make a right." However, a faulty premise or two notwithstanding, the Holistic Training Principle (again, which really should be renamed the "Experimentation Principle') is not *necessarily* wrong; experimentation per se is a good thing, as long as it is guided by rationality (we are reserving judgment, for now, concerning the rationality of volume training). On the other hand, the idea that training specifics should be dictated by instinct really just makes this idea a redundancy of the Instinctive Training Principle.

It is interesting that the inventor of this idea chose to differentiate between strength and mass training, since they are essentially one in the same. All things being equal, a bigger muscle is a stronger one, and vice-versa. Successful training, specifically for the purpose of strength, will produce the side-effect of increased muscle mass. Similarly, successfully training for mass requires that the subject become stronger. Many hold the view that training with a lower rep range and lower time under tension (total time it takes to complete a set) will result in greater strength, but viewed in the context of a bodybuilding regiment, it holds true that strength and size training are the same thing.

This principle also fails to define what is meant by "refinement" training, although the commonly-held view is that training with light weights for high repetitions will somehow "refine" or (to use the most overused and misunderstood term in the vocabulary of especially casual weight trainers) "tone" one's muscles. This view has no evidence or viable theory to support it, and it is contrary to what we know about the importance of intensity as it relates to the mechanism of adaptation to stress. A muscle can do three things: It can get bigger, it can get smaller, or it can stay the same size. There is one thing it cannot do: It cannot be "refined." The idea of refinement or "toning" also supposes that light training will have a localized fat-burning effect (otherwise known as spot reduction), which has been proven to be false.

In the last few days before a bodybuilding competition, a popular ploy among some competitors is repeatedly striking bodybuilding poses, contracting each muscle with all the energy he can muster. The idea is that, like "refinement" training, this method will harden the appearance of the muscles. This is a false notion. In all likelihood, the muscles will appear more flat as a result of this action, since muscular contraction reduces the glycogen levels of the muscles. Reduced glycogen levels will cause the muscle to have a more flat and flaccid appearance.

Progressive Overload Principle

The principle

The idea here is that in order to add muscle mass, the subject ought to progressively increase the amount of weight he is using for a certain number of repetitions, or increase the amount of repetitions he is able to perform with a certain weight, or both. For muscles to get bigger, they must get stronger, and vice-versa—so anyone wanting to put on size needs to concentrate on getting stronger.

Conclusions

It is a fact that the body must be subjected to ever-increasing levels of stress in order to adapt accordingly. It is true that if muscles are to be made bigger, they must also be made stronger. Although the use of the word "overload" is superfluous and adds a bit of confusion to the idea of progression, this principle is correct.

Pre-Exhaustion Training Principle

The principle

The idea behind pre-exhaustion is that the technique allows one to fully isolate, and therefore most productively train, a particular muscle. This is accomplished by training that body part first with a single-joint, direct isolation exercise so that the muscle becomes fatigued, or pre-exhausted, and then immediately proceeding to a heavier, compound-type movement. The benefit is that the effectiveness of the second exercise will not be limited by the capabilities of lesser, weaker muscles. We can use the example of a chest-training workout. The subject has opted to perform bench presses. The bench press is a good mass-building exercise because a large number of muscle fibers are used when performed properly. But often times failure will be reached because smaller muscles (such as the triceps) give out before the larger, target muscle (chest). This naturally limits the effectiveness of bench presses as a chest exercise. So in a pre-exhaustion set, the subject will first perform an isolation movement such as cable crossovers first, since this exercise isolates the chest and disinvolves the triceps.

Conclusions

Pre-Exhaustion is an effective remedy for the shortcomings of compound (multiple joint) exercises. It is a good tactic, and an idea espoused by both volume and high-intensity proponents.

Split System Training Principle

The principle

This method specifies that the subject should divide his workout regiment so that he trains only a certain number of body parts per session, rather than training the entire body in a single workout. The subject should arrange his training sessions so that they are spread out over multiple days.

Conclusions

This is a sensible and practical tactic. Other than those who are in the first week or two of weightlifting, it is essential to work the whole body over the span of several days, so that an optimum amount of energy can be devoted to each body part. Virtually everyone who trains seriously with weights uses this method, and for good reason.

Muscle Confusion Principle

The principle

In order to avoid stagnation and halted progress, the subject ought to "confuse" his muscles by changing exercises, number of sets and reps, or any other variables in his training regiment. This abrupt change will shock the body into growth, and progress will be resumed.

Conclusions

Progressive growth is a result of progression of intensity—that of continually applying greater and greater stress to the muscles being trained. One way to insure that greater and greater stress is applied over time is to keep as many variables as possible constant. An obvious example of an effort to reduce variables is training with the same exercises over an extended period of time. Since the exercises remain the same, the subject should then only concern himself with progressively lifting heavier weights, or performing more reps with the same weight (or both), since either progression constitutes an increase in stress.

This isn't to say that one should never change his training regiment. Sometimes it can be a good idea, as long as 1) the new, or any regiment, is given ample opportunity to manifest a progression of increasing stress, and 2) the new regiment represents an improvement over the old one. Change for the sake of change is not likely to produce much improvement. Sometimes a simple change can help avert burnout, so for this purpose it can be a good idea. Frequent change is almost certainly not good, since by definition there will be too many variables present to insure progression. As with all other components of a weight-training program, change should come about because of thoughtful analysis, not whims.

Finally, this is another case of a training tactic that is a bit of a misnomer. Muscles cannot become "confused." They experience stress, and they adapt accordingly. If they experience increasingly elevated stress, they will progressively adapt by growing.

Cycle Training Principle

The principle

Cycle training is a tactic whereby the subject will break his training into two or more parts, each executed over a fairly long term (usually three or more months). Each period will concentrate on a different type of training, with different expected results; these periods will variously concentrate on strength, mass, refinement, or whatever other type of training the subject desires. Each period will have its own unique recipe of exercises, number of sets and reps, tempo of workout, frequency, degrees of intensity, or whatever other variables that seem suitable for manipulation.

Conclusions

Considering all the flawed concepts that are rolled into this single tactic, I am tempted to wonder if any bad ideas were left out. This idea contains problems that have already been discussed with the Set System, Eclectic, Holistic, and Muscle Confusion principles.

Forced Reps Principle

Principle

Forced reps is a method whereby the subject is able to train beyond failure. After completing the last repetition that is possible under his own power, the subject will continue to lift the weight with the assistance of a helper or "spotter."

Conclusions

Using forced reps is a good way to train beyond failure, the idea being that the maximum intensity of stress possible will be experienced by the muscles being trained. As with the pre-exhaustion technique, it is a good tactic. It is also an idea espoused by both volume and high-intensity proponents.

Construction of a volume training theory

We should now revisit the question of whether the above principles collectively form a coherent theory. In their present form they do not. Again, and to their collective credit, they make no such pretense. At the same time, these principles have been often been presented as a "system," which to some might suggest an underlying theoretical coherency or at least orderly arrangement. This collection meets the criteria of neither, and it seems as though the principles raise more questions than they answer. Nevertheless, one might be able to extract and organize the collection's fundamental assertions in the hope that a workable volume training theory will be revealed or at least alluded to. Before attempting to do so, we ought to first make a clear delineation between the principles listed above, and what are advertised to be principles but are actually weight-training tactics. Having done so, the most sensible theory I was able to construct used the following four principles:

Set System Training

Instinctive Training

Holistic Training

Progressive Overload

These appear to be the only real principles in the lot, the rest being tactics. From this point forward, Instinctive Training will be referred to as "Intuitive Training" and Holistic Training as "Experimental Training" because left unchanged, especially in the case of the former, they are logically self-destructive. These principles are certainly the victims of careless nomination, although it should be noted that their independent cogency is not necessarily assured by simple renaming.

Using the four principles, here is the volume training theory I was able to construct:

1) Muscle mass can be increased by lifting weights for a certain number of sets for each exercise. The amount of muscle growth that will result from the weightlifting rises with the number of sets that are performed, *except* when:
    (a) The subject, through intuition, comes to possess knowledge about the ideal number of sets for maximum muscle growth, and adjusts his training accordingly, *or*
    (b) The subject, through experimentation, comes to possess this knowledge, and he changes his training to suit the discovery.
2) In order to continue properly stimulating growth, the subject ought to progressively increase the amount of weight he is lifting.

Before proceeding, it can be acknowledged that the second point is without question valid. It is logical and has been proven through experimentation. It is not inconsistent with any and all knowledge we possess of human physiology. It is also the one principle that is expressly shared by high-intensity and high-volume theory.

That being said, it is clear that this is a theory of sparse constructs—so it must be determined what was left out. To get a clearer picture of what is meant by this, imagine trying to explain the idea of lifting weights for the purpose of increasing muscle mass to an alien visitor, one with a physiology completely different from that of humans. Imagine explaining exactly why one event causes the other. The above explanation does not succeed in this regard, so it is therefore not a complete theory. A theory should not be predicated on assumptions, much like it should not be taken for granted that an alien visitor would even know that lifting weights builds bigger muscles. After all, evidently the prevalence of assumption is the reason for the very conspicuous absence of a complete volume training theory, since no one ever bothered to try to write one down—just as the prevalence of assumption at one time was responsible for everyone thinking that the Earth was flat.

Since the theory has holes in it, it's important to define exactly what the assumptions or missing premises of the current theory are, describe their relevance to the theory, and arrange them so that the theory can be made complete. Whenever possible, it should be considered appropriate to draw upon scientifically accepted knowledge of human physiology and weight-training to fill these holes. There are four hypothetical principles that appear to be missing and assumed:

Frequency: Sufficient rest should occur between workouts.

Special Intensity: Workouts must be performed with sufficient intensity and duration.

Physiological Disparity: Everyone has a unique physiology and unique demands.

Special Adaptation: The body responds to the stress of exercise by building muscle.

Below is a description of each idea, its role within the theory, and whatever problems each might create:

Frequency

The theory does not specify training frequency or the need for rest days, or how many days should pass between workouts. Rather, the theory apparently assumes that rest days will take place between workouts, especially since volume training regiments always prescribe a certain number of these days (and also due to a passing reference to rest days in the Intuitive Training Principle). We can further imagine that the subject, remaining with the guidelines of volume training theory, can modify this number by invoking the Intuitive or Experimental principles. Although a certain number of rest days is not defined, it is clearly assumed that one should rest for an appropriate amount of time between workouts so that repair and growth can take place. This is a valid and necessary idea.

Special Intensity

As in the case with Frequency, intensity of effort is an implied principle of volume training, because a few high-intensity tactics are mentioned above. It seems to be further suggested that all non-warm up sets should be performed with a high or maximum level of intensity. This idea is consistent with what we know about the body's adaptive system responding in proportion to the intensity of stress, not the duration. However, since by definition a volume training regiment includes a large number of sets, the body's ability to generate intensity will decrease throughout the workout, and duration then becomes an important factor. The volume training Intensity Principle therefore implies that 1) a second mechanism separate from the body's adaptation mechanism is at work here, or 2) there might be a peculiar attribute of the body's adaptation mechanism—and that both respond to duration of stress as well as intensity. Furthermore, this mechanism must apply to muscular contraction only (since similar attributes have yet to be observed in the body's response to any other types of stress; in other words, the degree of the body's response to all other forms of stress is dependent upon intensity only, and never upon duration). Neither has ever been discovered. This is the first major problem with volume training theory.

Physiological Disparity

A certain number of sets per body part or exercise is not specified by the volume training theory, only that there should be "multiple" sets. On top of that, there is a large disparity between the number of sets recommended by different volume training proponents—and an equally large difference between the numbers of sets performed by the volume trainers themselves. When it is also factored in that one should consult the Intuitive and Experimental principles in order to formulate an optimal, personal training regiment, we are forced to deduce that everyone has unique physiological demands and indeed, a unique physiology, and that no number of sets is ideal for everyone—thus a training regiment must be tailored to suit each individual. This idea is in stark contrast to the Identity Principle specified in high-intensity theory. It is also in direct opposition to the findings of the medical sciences over the last several centuries. Every human is genetically unique, but we all have the same basic physiological makeup and functions. If there is evidence to the contrary, the medical sciences community would be quite interested to learn of this discovery. But there is no such evidence. Rather, there is limitless evidence that humans share a uniform physiology. This is the second major problem with the theory.

Special Adaptation

There must be a mechanism whereby the act of lifting weights will somehow translate into an increase in muscle mass. In other words, the body must adapt to the stress of intense muscular contractions (and/or longer-duration contractions, per the "Intensity" principle listed above) by creating an adaptation, in this case building bigger muscles. The general adaptation syndrome has already been explained. And the adaptive mechanism stated in the assumed Special Intensity Principle implies that the idea that the body responds in kind to the intensity of stress is not a complete one, and that something is missing: The body either needs a set-counting mechanism or a mechanism that somehow responds to lower-intensity, higher-duration muscular contractions, and that this mechanism should be unique to the stress of muscular contractions, since it has been observed in no other types of stress. On top of that, since we know that low-volume, high-intensity training, performed properly, can and will cause a significant increase in muscle mass, this physiological feature would be a redundancy. The problem here is essentially identical to the problem with the Special Intensity Principle.

Concerning the idea of a mechanism for growth apart from G.A.S. that would make multiple-set training beneficial, some are quick to point out that the accumulation of microtrauma (the actual tearing of muscle fibers during a workout) from set to set will have the effect of greater growth. If this were the case, for maximum growth, *very* long workouts should be prescribed, since it is reasonable to assume that microtrauma will accumulate, and the more sets performed, the more microtrauma will take place. However, it is also reasonable to imagine that the degree of microtrauma that should occur will be dependent upon the intensity of stress inflicted upon the muscles, and that especially among advanced lifters whose muscles have become resistant to microtrauma, the amount of microtrauma that will occur will drop off sharply as the intensity of stress decreases.

And just like training itself, there can very easily be too much of a good thing. Regardless of the amount of microtrauma that actually takes place, a single high-intensity set has been proven to be able to stimulate growth, and creating microtrauma in excess of this might be highly detrimental; greater recovery periods will be required, and in some cases, high levels of microtrauma can actually kill muscle cells and invite injury. Also, there is some disagreement about the amount of real benefit that will result from inducing microtrauma.[12] The observed repair of microtrauma by the body has led some to assume that this action is the mechanism for muscular growth, whereas there might be reason to be believe that it is nothing more than simple localized damage control.

Volume training theory conclusions

We could further question the idea of using intuition or unguided experimentation to fine-tune the volume training regiment, but at this point that might just be adding insult to injury. In the spirit of scientific method, I was not able to construct a viable theory for volume-oriented weight-training. It appears that the only thing that could rescue the idea is the discovery of a couple of human physiological attributes that would impact far more than the small world of weigh training. Indeed, if anyone were to prove the existence of the Physiological Disparity and Special Adaptation principles, that person could clear a space on his mantle for a Nobel Prize. As such, volume training will remain a hypothesis. It is not a cogent theory.

But despite all of this, for some, volume training works. *How can this be?*

Why volume training works (for some)

Volume training is fairly unique in that it is an example of a theory that has fatal cogency but can, at times, stand up to empirical observation. Why is this? In *Heavy Duty,* Mentzer admitted that the physiques of many champions are "in part" the result of volume training, but that they were more likely to have built a good deal of their mass using lower-volume work.[13] This seems to be a little dismissive, and for the most part, not true. A lot of champions have never used anything *but* volume training. This begs an important question: How can volume training work?

It seems as if there really can be only one answer, and it is very simple: Volume training is an approximation of high-intensity training. It is a *clumsy* approximation, but an approximation nonetheless. High-intensity training theory is reflected through volume training, though in a very imprecise manner—and hidden within any volume training session *is* a high-intensity workout. In nearly all volume training workouts (just like in the high-intensity strategy), the subject performs one high or maximum-intensity set for each exercise. But then he performs a lot of other sets too. Apart from the single set that by itself was sufficient to stimulate growth, the other sets are meaningless, although they have five effects. These extra sets will:

1. Burn extra calories.
2. Break down muscle and/or connective tissue further.
3. Create greater general recovery demands.
4. Subtract from the intensity and effectiveness of the remaining exercises.
5. Increase the risk of injury.

Without question extra sets burn more calories. For this reason, quite a few bodybuilders make the mistake of training with even greater volume before a contest, the thinking being that this will contribute to their fat-burning efforts. But as mentioned in the analysis of the "Eclectic Training Principle," it is an infinitely better idea to clearly divide mass and fat-burning training.

Point four should not be taken lightly. Just about all workouts ?˙ comprised of multiple exercises, and the majority of workouts ˙

training more than one body part. If quite a few exercises are performed for the first body part, with multiple sets for each taken to or beyond failure, then it should be expected that the amount of intensity the subject is able to devote to each set will diminish as the workout proceeds. It should be the primary aim of anyone committing to bodybuilding to build an even, balanced physique. It should be rather difficult to achieve this if the effort one is able to devote to certain body parts will be impaired.

Regarding points two and three, it should be noted that one major factor determining the amount of muscle that can be added by any given subject is his ability to quickly recover from exercise. This appears to be even more critical a factor for the volume-trained bodybuilder, since there is far more recovering to do. Although the subject has sufficiently stimulated growth, he continues to train, and every set after the first will subtract from the desired effect, that of increased muscle mass—since the drain on the body is cumulative. To illustrate this point, the following graphs have been constructed to show the cumulative effectiveness of a single training session:

GRAPH 1

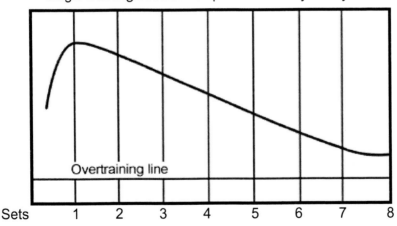

Cumulative hypothetical effectiveness of a
single training session: Superior recovery ability

(↑ Muscular growth resulting from a single exercise)

GRAPH 2

Cumulative hypothetical effectiveness of a
single training session: Inferior recovery ability

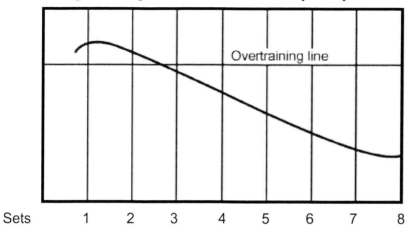

Sets   1   2   3   4   5   6   7   8

The curved line represents the overall hypothetical effectiveness of the training session. The workout becomes less and less effective as it drags on. The training session can be concluded and considered effective as long as the accumulated damage and drain on the body's resources do not plunge below the overtraining line (assuming that enough rest will occur before the next workout for that body part). These graphs assume that the subject is able to achieve the highest level of intensity on the first working set. In reality, a second set might have a higher intensity level, in which case the bottom-line effectiveness of a workout might peak with that set—although the extra recovery required by the second set might negate the increase. Even if high levels of intensity can be maintained throughout the workout (which they can't), the overall effectiveness of the workout will steadily head south due to the accumulating recovery requirements. Stimulation is not cumulative. Damage is.

The ability of the volume-trained bodybuilder to grow in spite of the inefficiency and counterproductivity of this approach is a function of his elevated physiological ability to mostly withstand the increased damage of redundant efforts. It appears that such an ability is unusual, considering the disparity between the vast number of bodybuilding hopefuls employing a volumistic approach, and the very few that are able to realize muscular mass of the first order. It's reasonable to deduce that this range of ability would also serve to widen the chasm between the genetically gifted few (and/or those that have opted for chemical enhancement)—some of whom seem to grow almost no matter how they train—and those with an average or inferior genetic ability for recovery, since the non-*ubermensch* types, by copying the champions, are destined to fail. Such individuals would give themselves a much better chance of achieving growth by employing high-intensity training (since proper recover time is an absolute requisite), rather than the volume method (which was born of the same physio-mythological parent that tends to advise fewer days of rest), which has historically under-rated or even ignored the importance of avoiding overtraining.

One theoretical advantage of volume training is that the subject is able to make several attempts with every exercise to generate the highest possible intensity. With strict high-intensity training, there can be no second chances (although it is not unheard-of in a high-intensity workout to perform a second set if the subject was not properly motivated to execute the first with optimum intensity). The second-chances idea is attractive, but with volume training, as the workout proceeds and the body becomes fatigued, the chance of elevating the intensity level of any given set is increasingly reduced. But the body *will* respond to whichever set creates the most stress. The question is whether this advantage outweighs the negative effect of performing multiple sets. If one is able to achieve optimum or highest intensity with the first set, as should be the case, then the answer is an unqualified no.

But it is reasonable to imagine that the best, most intense set might occasionally come after the first. So the question is that of simple return-on-investment: Will the benefits of performing additional sets, where increased intensity is achieved, outweigh the cost of additional recovery requirements? This will depend on two factors:

1. The difference in quality (i.e. the level of intensity) between the first set and a later, better set, and
2. The individual's recovery ability.

Since for our purposes it's not really possible to tell if it is worth it to perform more sets in the hope of performing a better one as the workout proceeds, it should be in the interest of the subject to master the motivational angle of his training efforts, so that when the time comes, he will be able to produce all-out exertion for a single, highly productive set. One added benefit of this approach is that in so doing, he can help avoid what is possibly the greatest pitfall of them all: Injury.

Volume and injury

After more than a quarter century of weightlifting, I have successfully avoided serious injury—and this might just be the single most attractive benefit of high-intensity training. Volume training can excessively damage muscular tissue and wear down joints; combined with inadequate recovery time, a small and unnoticeable injury can eventually turn into a nuisance or in the worst cases, a disablement (such as an acute severe injury like a complete muscle tear). In some cases, the ultimate result will be a capitulation of the effort in its entirety: Deprived of ability to continue training as before, the bodybuilder will quit lifting weights altogether, and all the time and energy spent will be forever lost—and there are few things more tragic.

Granted, high-intensity trained bodybuilders are not impervious to injury, as evidenced by Dorian Yates' 1994 biceps tear (although he was performing an exercise that is particularly dangerous for that muscle, p.143). Indeed, lifting any type of heavy weight, regardless of the style of training or precision of execution, involves the possibility of injury. In the absence of any scientific study to specifically compare the rate and severity of weight-training injuries for the purpose of assessing the relative safety of the two styles in question, it may be necessary to make judgments based on personal experience and through observing the experiences of others—and these observations have confirmed the supposition that the excessive wear-and-tear of volume training results in more (and more serious) injuries.

But in addition to these anecdotes, a study comparing rates of injury between powerlifters and bodybuilders provides some evidence to support this assertion. In his article entitled "Minimizing Weight Training Injuries in Bodybuilders and Athletes," first published in *Topics in Clinical Chiropractic,* Ben Weitz, DC, noted the following:

Many weight training injuries may be related to stressing the same joints repeatedly until muscular or tendinous failure occurs. Repeatedly training to failure without any periodization or cycling of the intensity or duration of the workouts increases the risk of tendinitis and other injuries. So, too, does the large volume and frequency of training.[14]

He further noted:

...there is some evidence that power lifters and Olympic lifters may actually have a slightly lower rate of injuries than bodybuilders. For example, despite using much heavier weight in the bench press than bodybuilders, power lifters seem to have a lower incidence of pectoralis major tears. Reynolds and colleagues (who performed the study) concluded that part of the problem was the total volume of work that bodybuilders perform.[15]

What makes this conclusion most compelling is Weitz's description of a typical amount of volume involved with a normal bodybuilding subject's training:

...it would not be unusual for a bodybuilder to perform five different exercises for his or her chest with four to five sets of each exercise using 6 to 15 repetitions. At least two or three of these sets will typically be taken to *failure* (ie, the point at which no more repetitions [reps] can be performed). Advanced techniques are also often employed. These techniques include forced reps, cheating reps, drop the weight sets, negatives, and supersets.[16]

In the higher-volume subjects mentioned in the above paragraph, Weitz describes a workout in which up to 15 sets are taken to, or beyond, failure. I have personally witnessed bodybuilders performing double this.

That there is a greater incidence of injury among these people should come as no surprise to anyone. My current chest routine consists of taking a total of two sets beyond failure: One set of Smith machine inclines, and one set of Hammer Strength decline presses. That's it: Two sets—and the results have been very good. Despite the fact that I will rest as many as ten days between each chest workout, I often feel as though I would be overtrained if I were to perform more sets.

Of course I perform a decent number of warm-up sets, as this is absolutely essential for avoiding injury. As a side note, although these are stopped far short of failure, I think to the casual observer they cloak the fact that I am actually performing a very small number of actual working sets. But for any given body part, I do not ever perform more actual total sets than can be counted on one hand, in fact I average three. I have built, and over a very long time, maintained a fairly high degree of muscle mass. And since I switched to the high-intensity style of training a great many years ago, I have been injury-free.

It's easy to imagine that the accumulation of wear-and-tear will contribute to a higher rate of injury among volume versus high-intensity trainers, especially considering that high-intensity training by itself does not imply the use of very heavy weights, as is the case with powerlifting. In fact, the amount of weight used by the low and high-volume camps is not significantly different. Volume trainers with excellent recovery abilities are sometimes quite strong. But a clear and objective way to compare the risk of injury between the two styles can be based on a simple comparison of the amount of training itself, or the sheer amount of opportunity for injury.

An injury can come at any time, during any set. My two-set chest workout, apart from obviously being very low volume, is also very infrequent: I train chest about once every nine days. To contrast this, quite a few bodybuilders that perform about 20 working sets for chest. Of these, let's suppose that half are so-called "finishing" movements such as dumbbell and machine flies. These exercises tend to involve fewer muscle fibers and less weight, so the risk of injury with each is low. We will therefore eliminate these from the comparison. The volume trainers are now left with ten sets per workout that carry a risk of injury. And since many of these people train on a four-on, one-off split, we can calculate the following: Supposing that all subjects in this example (my own workout included as the high-intensity version) take a total of one month off from training over the course of a year, here are the total number of workouts and sets performed during that year:

High-intensity: 36 training sessions, 72 sets

Volume training: 66 training sessions, 660 sets

We can see that the volume trainer has more than nine times the opportunity to suffer major injury (in this case, a pectoral tear) than his high-intensity counterpart. This does not even take into account the greater predisposition to injury that the volume trainer carries due to wear-and-tear. This wear-and-tear will often manifest itself in the less dramatic but equally disabling rotator cuff injury, a common occurrence. Studies measuring rate of injury among athletes and bodybuilders include both muscle tears and various rotator cuff problems, and a host of other occurrences. What is most telling about these studies is the simple fact that they almost always reflect the number of injuries per hours of activity. In 1995 and again in 2000, for example, there were 2.6 injuries reported per 1000 hours of activity.[17] As incredible as it may sound, there are some volume trainers that exercise as many as 1000 hours in a single year. Since wear-and-tear is cumulative, these people (or those training even half as often) should consider major injury to be an eventuality.

For someone with an unrelenting desire to be a success in bodybuilding, would not a complete muscle tear be a horrible nightmare? These tears require immediate surgery, long layoff and rehabilitation periods, and the torn muscle is very rarely returned to its previous state— not to mention the huge hospital bills if the victim does not have good medical insurance. Despite the nonexistent theoretical foundation of volume training, and faced with evidence that high-intensity training is effective, some people forever refuse to forsake the volume approach. But forget the logic. Forget the proof. If there is just one reason why bodybuilders should at least try high-intensity training, this is it: It is safer.

Overtraining

Overtraining is physical state whereby the physiological recovery required by exercise exceeds the body's ability to recover. The graph on page 65 illustrates this phenomenon. Simply put, you are overtrained if you work out too much. A high-intensity set will stimulate growth, but it will also cause an acute breakdown of muscular tissue and a general drain on the body's resources. Volume trainers perform a single high-intensity set that stimulates growth, but then they make the mistake of performing a large number of additional sets, thinking that the result will be more growth.

The total stimulative effect of the entire workout cannot exceed the stimulation achieved by the most intense single set. There is no cumulative effect of stimulation. However, there most certainly is an accumulation of acute damage. Long weightlifting workouts are draining, and there are limited resources available within the body to compensate for this. Overtraining manifests itself when the subject begins his next training session before his recovery has been completed.

When overtraining occurs, all progress is halted. In fact, overtraining will cause regression, because the body is never even given a chance to return to the state it was in prior to the workout. The subject will actually *lose* mass. Obviously this is something that everyone training with weights should seek to avoid. Nevertheless, overtraining is the single most common pitfall among bodybuilders. This issue is mentioned in the volume training chapter because it is a physical state that is almost exclusively the domain of volume trainers, for two reasons:

1. Volume trainers, by definition, perform a large number of sets.
2. High-intensity training theory mandates adequate recovery time.

Any subject performing a large volume of training should expect that he will become overtrained at some point. Some individuals appear to be constantly overtrained, but one might be left to suppose that these people are so familiar, even comfortable, with their overtrained state that they fail to recognize that anything is wrong—other than that they never make any progress. The tendency in these cases seems to be to blame other variables, genetics topping the list.

Academic discussions of overtraining typically center on a generally overtrained condition, whereby the body's resources are not adequate to restore the body to its pre-workout condition, and are certainly not adequate for growth on top of repair. There further might exist the peril of acute overtraining. The intense contractions of a weight-training workout actually tear muscle fibers. This action is known as *microtrauma*. Training the same muscle before it has been given adequate time to recover from this damage will insure, quite obviously, that it will not progress (although there is some disagreement on this point; see p. 83): The higher the volume of training, the greater the accumulation of damage.

A thoughtful, deliberate training regiment that seeks to efficiently apply the science of mass-building should by design steer the subject clear of overtraining. Nevertheless, it is important to be aware of the signs of overtraining, which apart from the inevitable losses in strength and size, may include the following[18]:

1. General fatigue
2. Persistent muscle soreness
3. Joint soreness
4. Elevated heart rate
5. Irritability
6. Loss of motivation
7. Depression
8. Insomnia
9. Loss of appetite
10. Weight loss
11. Decreased sex drive
12. Susceptibility to infection or disease

Anyone that comes to the realization that he is overtrained needs to immediately take some time off, otherwise his condition will deteriorate. It is generally agreed that two weeks is sufficient for allowing the body to recharge and repair itself. During this time the subject should perform zero weightlifting workouts. However, light cardio is advisable, as it will keep the metabolism from slowing down during the break. The subject also ought to spend some time analyzing his training, since obviously he has been overdoing it somewhere, or maybe even everywhere. Upon his return, he should have made changes to his regiment thus that he might avoid returning to this overtrained state.

Volume and prioritization

Brief mention was made in the section *Why volume training works (for some)* of the point that long, volume-oriented workouts will necessarily cause the subject to favor certain body parts and exercises over others, since intensity levels *will* drop off as a workout proceeds; some body parts will be trained later in the workout than others, and these will necessarily fall victim to lower intensity. And as we have seen, suboptimal intensity will create suboptimal results. In other words, the development of whichever body parts are trained first will benefit, and those trained last (or really, whichever body parts are not trained first) will suffer. With competitive bodybuilders this can be a rather large problem, since it should be their goal to create the most perfectly balanced physique possible.

Many volume trainers have sought to remedy this problem by using double- or even triple-splits, so that body parts that would otherwise be de-prioritized could be trained with greater intensity. Body parts that would ordinarily be trained second or third, by using splits, can be trained first in subsequent sessions, after leaving the gym and then returning after a few hours have passed. Indeed, this will allow the subject to train these body parts harder.

However, anyone that feels it is necessary to visit the gym twice in one day is almost certainly training too much in the first place. Additionally, the extra intensity accrued from multiple daily visits, compounded with the already high volume, will push the subject closer to (or deeper into) an overtrained state. And typically, when using a double-split, the subject will further increase volume. On top of all this, visiting the gym too frequently will often, by itself, help induce a state of mental burnout—even if the subject is somehow able to avert physical burnout. And after all, this is the key variable: The idea that the subject will somehow avoid overtraining, despite the high volume and frequent gym visits. All too often the subject *is* overtrained—and in those cases, the question of which body parts and exercises the subject is able to devote more intensity to is therefore moot. Only in the rarest of cases can a subject employ high volume and multiple daily visits and not be overtrained.

In contrast, high-intensity training sessions are, by nature, short enough to allow for high levels of intensity throughout their duration. And since the low-volume approach all but guarantees that each body part and exercise can be trained with optimum intensity, one can expect to achieve even and complete development by using it (anomalous genetic deficiencies notwithstanding). For many, even and complete development is the name of the game. Double-splits are not necessary, and are in fact not advisable. And who has time for that anyway?

Investment of time

One more thing is worth pointing out: Without question, high-intensity training is time-efficient. I neither have the time or inclination to blunder my way through long, volume-oriented workouts, so the brief and infrequent nature of the high-intensity approach makes it that much more attractive. I am often asked how many hours per day I spend in the gym. There are a good deal of misconceptions held by the general public about bodybuilding, and the amount of time that one must devote to the undertaking is near the top of the list. This being the case, most expect me to say as little as two or as many as five. When I tell them that I never spend more than an hour, the reaction is typically disbelief. Actually, for some workouts I am able to get it down to under 40 minutes, but this means no talking or waiting for machines.

Apart from the large investment of time the volume trainer must make, many fall victim to severe burnout or injury and end up quitting for good, with volume training itself as the likely culprit. Many volume trainers spend a good deal more than ten hours a week in the gym, but for the sake of example, let's suppose that such an investment of time is normal. Many high-intensity trainers spend far less than four, but again, we'll use this number for our comparison. So that's six extra hours per week spent in the gym for the volume-trainer. Assuming once more that each subject takes a full month off per year, the volume-trainer must devote an extra 288 hours, during the course of that year, to the gym. A fair number of bodybuilders make money as personal trainers. Imagine if the extra 288 hours were devoted to training clients at $50/hour (many trainers charge a good deal more). That's an extra $14,400 that could have been earned during that year.

And if you consider the case of the severe burnout or injury victim that at one point leaves the gym for the last time, never to return, all the time spent is forever lost. As many of these people, after a relatively short while, return to a level of appearance such that no one would ever guess that they once were avid bodybuilders (this *does happen*), then all the time spent is truly lost. Actually, many are worse-off, since it is often the case that they must live with the injuries they incurred through weightlifting for the rest of their lives.

Many quit after as many as ten years of devoted training, some a good deal more. We can thus consider the following time spent in the gym: If we imagine 10 hours per week, times 48 weeks out of the year (four weeks off), times 10 years, we can see that 4800 hours have been lost forever. If you factor in extra time spent preparing for, and traveling to and from the gym, this can easily add an extra 800 hours over the span of ten years. And these are all *conservative* numbers! For some, the number can be as high as 10,000 hours over ten years. Think of what could have been accomplished otherwise had the subject known that all would be for naught. And this does not even take into account the large amount of money the bodybuilder is almost certain to have spent on gym memberships, supplements, workout apparel, etc.

Strategy Conclusions

For every effect there is a cause. Nothing ever happens "just because." There is a viable scientific theory regarding why stress in the form of exercise can have the effect of increasing muscle mass. It is a fairly simple cause-and-effect relationship. High-intensity training was devised as means to apply this knowledge in the most efficient and effective manner possible. The volume trained subject adds muscular mass due to precisely the same science as his high-intensity counterpart. However, high volume training was not devised to be an optimum application of this knowledge, since the volume training idea predates any attempt to create a cogent scientific theory for muscle-building. Likewise, the idea of the Universe being structured so that the Earth is at its center was never meant to be an application of the modern science of astronomy, because again, the idea predated the scientific knowledge. But at the time it seemed like a good idea, and there was even some evidence supporting it. The same thing could be said for volume training.

In the end, we can give some credit to volume training because, despite a lack of theoretical foundation, it was able to come reasonably close to an ideal type of training. Some of what was learned and eventually became the "principles" of volume training surely came about from simple trial-and-error. But as mentioned, for muscular growth there are two factors that make a trial-and-error approach very difficult:

1. Muscle growth comes about very slowly.
2. There are a large number of variables in the equation.

The variables that can affect the outcome of a physical exercise cause-and-effect experiment include nutrition, amount of rest, supplements, emotional state, other physical activity, and general health, to name a few. Trying to control all of them over a long enough timeline to notice conclusive results would be problematic. The difficulty in controlling variables might be the reason for ideas like *giant sets* being accepted as effective. In fact, many of the accepted "principles" (tactics) of the volume training recipe are just plain wrong. They were unguided and theoretically unsupported guesses, but apparently seemed to be neat ideas—and the negative results of experiments with them, if there *were* any, were apparently never fully revealed, lost amongst all the variables the subject encountered over the duration of the experiment.

But almost certainly there weren't any controlled experiments that created these ideas. It's reasonable to assume that the inventors of many of the tactics associated with volume training, above and beyond the familiar more-is-better mantra, just plain felt that *hard work will pay off, no matter what you do*. Without question, giant sets are hard. Try to do four or five exercises in row for a single body part, exerting as much effort as humanly possible for each portion—with no rest between exercises. Now repeat that four times. It's very tough, and very tiring. And it's counterproductive.

In the vast clutter of variables to be considered, it can be difficult to determine which tactic is productive and which is not, especially since we can image a great multitude of tactics being used in a single regiment. Tactics without theoretical foundation can easily be misconstrued one way or another. But with the volume training compilation of tactics, there seems to be an "anything is worth trying" attitude. I credit the inventors for their optimism!

As a system, the effectiveness of volume training for a select few is why it has been misconstrued by many as optimal, and it is why some will suppose or assume that it has an independent theoretical basis. As I hope to have proven, it does not. But it does work for some people, and there is a very real, scientific reason for why it does—which happens to be exactly the same reason that high-intensity training works. They are both applications of the same science. And it is in this application of the science of mass-building that volume training loses its way. In fact, it is an unwitting application, because volume training does not recognize the existence of its own scientific underpinnings. It appears to have been formulated in a rather blind fashion, and as one might guess with any such formulation, the method has a few problems. The end result is that volume training, when compared to high-intensity, is less efficient and less effective.

This begs a very obvious question: Does this mean that champion bodybuilders (or anyone, really) that use volume training would have even better physiques if they used high-intensity training? There really can be only one answer: Yes, it most certainly does. The degree of the difference between the physique of the volume trained bodybuilder and what his physique *could have been* if his training had been of the high-intensity variety is dependent upon two factors:

1. His recovery ability.
2. The specifics of his training regiment.

In the case of an individual with excellent recovery ability who, although training in a volume-oriented style, keeps his sets moderate (say 12 sets instead of 20 per body part), then the difference between his physique and his *potential physique* will likely not be astronomical. However, an individual with poor recovery ability that performs a very high volume of work (I see these people every day) is very much selling himself short. Many of these people never seem to add a single ounce of muscle. With high-intensity training, at least they would be giving themselves a chance.

So am I saying that volume afficianados like Lee Haney and Arnold Schwarzenegger, or any number of volume training professionals, could have been better had they used high-intensity training? Without hesitation, my answer is yes (or maybe in some cases, the volume-trained bodybuilder could have reached top form more quickly). Although one should expect some to cry blasphemy, here is something worthy of consideration: Anyone following bodybuilding during the late 1980s should recall the absolute dominance of Haney. He worked very hard and had excellent genetics. He was competing against a field that all trained in the same style, more or less. Like Haney, they were volume trainers. It's certain that they all worked very hard as well.

It was Haney's incredible genetics that set him apart from crowd and made him the best bodybuilder in the world for eight straight years. In his last year of competing in the Mr. Olympia contest, Haney edged-out a fast-rising competitor from England named Dorian Yates, who used the high-intensity approach. One could argue that Haney had better genetics than Yates, but somehow, over the next few years, Yates was able to blow past the physique that had given Haney cause for alarm in his final contest. Whereas the mainly stagnant standard of mass for the prior eight years had been, on average, 245 pounds for the 5'11" Haney (at the time considered to be incredibly, even ultimately massive), within two years Yates was 257 pounds at 5'10"—with a level of conditioning that exceeded anything Haney had ever produced.

It didn't have to be this way. Yates could have been a volume trainer. With his genetics and determination, it's certain that he would have done very well—but it's debatable whether he would have risen above also-ran status, and he probably never would have become Mr. Olympia. And if this were the case, maybe we would now be answering the same question about him: "Do you really think that Yates would be *better* if he used high-intensity training?" Well, he *did* use high-intensity training, and he *was* better. And there was a time when he was clearly the best in the world. Some will charge that this is a naïve viewpoint, and that the difference in physiques amounted to better genes and especially better drugs, not better training. Even if that were the case, within a few years it can be imagined that the playing field had been leveled. Yates nevertheless continued to prevail, and was undefeated for the next half decade.

And from my personal experience, I can say that my physique improved dramatically once I made the switch from volume to high-intensity training. Although I do not have an Olympian-caliber physique, I cannot possibly imagine that I would have been able to build as good of a physique through volume training. I have also had tremendous longevity, as the nature of brief and infrequent training has kept me from becoming injured or mentally burned out.

That being said, after a fairly exhaustive analysis, the following conclusions have been reached about volume training:

1. No theoretical foundation
2. Works for some
3. Time-consuming
4. Energy-consuming
5. Greatly elevated risk of injury
6. Greatly elevated risk of overtraining
7. Less effective

Clearly, the approach leaves much to be desired.

Personal observations

It seems clear that slight increases in mass through drawn-out, moderate stress activities have helped foster the volume training mentality—which has thus made further remote and counterintuitive the idea of intensity of stress dictating muscle growth. An example would be the slight increase in leg mass enjoyed by soccer players, the (erroneous though common) idea being that the more one plays soccer, the bigger his legs will become. I consider myself to have exceptional leg development, and I continue to be amazed by the number of people that ask me if I got them as a result of soccer or even running. This flimsy association was even perpetrated by one of my own family members—when as a teenager, upon seeing that I had started lifting weights, my grandmother suggested that a better use of my time would be getting a job as a grocery bagger, since apart from generating income and supposedly enhancing my character, it would "build up" my muscles! Even at my young age I knew something was fishy about that statement.

So why don't all bodybuilders use high-intensity training? From my experience, most people don't know about it, experienced bodybuilders and weightlifters included. A few have heard about high-intensity training, and some have even read an article on the topic, but the idea is often dismissed as nonsense. As the Dorian Yates era continues to fade into memory, high-intensity training has not nearly reached the popularity or level of respect it deserves. With the apparent absence of a top-notch, serious and current competitor—with the physique to back it up—to carry the torch, and the prevailing crop (at least from what I have seen) mainly touting the volume approach, this is to be expected. Then again, with the state of men's professional bodybuilding becoming increasingly abominable (circa 2008), it's unlikely that the training strategy of any top competitor would have much influence. The current situation sort of reminds me of the cold war, where the superpowers would stockpile massive arsenals of nuclear weapons. A subtle metaphor of such mutual assured destruction is seen in men's professional bodybuilding, which in appearance now seems nothing more than an escalating battle of heavy chemical enhancement. (Maybe it's for the best that among that group there is no outspoken proponent of high-intensity training theory—lest people who don't know any better should run from it for fear of setting off a runaway process that will result in such a physique!) So the method remains largely unknown.

Of a legion of bodybuilders and weightlifters I have known over the years, many of whom I have had at least casual discussions about training methodology, almost no one has ever heard of Arthur Jones. A few have heard of Mike Mentzer. The majority know who Dorian Yates is, although not a great number are aware that his physique was the result of high-intensity training. But, as the world's top professional for half a decade, he was the idea's greatest ambassador—in a way that Jones could never have approximated, because of the obvious association of the application of the method and the results; Yates used high-intensity style training, and he was the best in the world; Jones, the mastermind, could only have limited influence, considering the combination of the apparent strangeness of his ideas and his relative lack of physical build. But apart from the near-invisibility of HIT, the volume style is so commonplace, and its apparent logic so deeply ingrained, that only a fraction of those using it are aware the term "volume training" exists at all!

I have also heard the incredible argument that high-intensity training is "too intellectual" in nature to be a worthwhile and effective system. (I suppose that the same thing could be said for an explanation of thermodynamics.) I am inclined to think that part of the reasoning here is that *a dumb activity ought to have a dumb system to support it.* I further reckon that part of the resistance against high-intensity training comes from a lack of understanding of its principles or scientific method in general. One can convey—with whatever degree of sophistication he desires—the rationale for high-intensity, low volume training. As one might expect, with any cross-section of avid gym-goers, sophisticated language is apt to leave a few in the dust.

But the actual workouts are exceedingly simple. One could approach such a regiment with precisely the same degree of examination commonly given to a volume-oriented system (little or none), and through proper execution, reap its benefits without the burden of immersing himself in intellectual discussions that, let's face it, are often out of place in bodybuilding circles anyway. Assuming that he is aware of the high-intensity approach, but unaware of or dumbfounded by the literature espousing it, our subject is then left to choose between it and volume training. Everyone I can think of that falls into this category chooses volume training, mainly because of what is little more than the draw of tradition, but also because of the faulty logic of context-switching (more hours in the office will yield greater returns; more hours in the gym should apparently do the same; the context has merely been switched).

And let's face it, for some, volume training works. Despite the redundancy of their training and associated negative effects, they grow nevertheless. I do see a much larger number that don't grow, however, and have spent years stuck at the same level of development. But if you are among those that have faith in volume training, you like it, it works for you, you have the time and energy for it, and you are okay with the elevated risk of injury, then by all means use it! I happily encourage those that are loyal to the idea to continue following it.

I found it immensely liberating once I came to the realization that a much better alternative to volume training was available. I will admit occasionally feeling a bit of anger over the excess time lost in gyms during my early phase. This tends to pass quickly, replaced by the satisfaction of righting a wrong. Also, in my volume training heyday, the decision to spend all that time in the gym was mine alone—and what does one stand to gain by staying angry at himself?

As for my early days of volume training, I do have to say that the amount of time and energy spent in the gym suited my enthusiasm. I was both obsessive and compulsive about it; I loved being in the gym, and looked forward to it with unabated enthusiasm—until I began to dread it. I was one of those people whose results from volume training had clear limitations. After a couple years of such training, maybe less, I began to go through a series of what I now know were overtrained periods. Around the same time I became aware of low-volume high-intensity training, but I was still young, unwise, and unsure. To me, high-intensity, low-volume training made sense. A regiment involving adequate recover time made sense. But the decent amount of progress I had made up to that point through volume training kept me clinging to that style. I had been sufficiently reinforced. However, the stagnated progress and desire for improvement prompted me to extinguish the old reinforcement and make some changes.

With some trepidation, I gradually started reducing my total sets. I discarded redundant exercises. But trusting, really believing that you can and will make that one set count is a necessity. It took me some time to get to that point. In addition to this, I began to train less frequently—from twice a week for each body part during the first couple of years to a three-on-one-off split for another couple, to four-on-one-off and then, by about the eighth year of my training, to a once-a-week system. It was when I became experienced and familiar with what I was capable of on a consistent basis that I finally ventured into very low volume training, using very infrequent training sessions. I've been training for about 24 years now, and for about the past seven I have had excellent results by training each body part as little as three times a month.

Progressive mechanical load training

One other strategy of training is worthy of mention: Progressive mechanical load training, better-known as Hypertrophy-Specific Training, or HST. Developed by Brian Haycock (who trademarked the HST name), it is very seldom used and is therefore not a part of the primary discussion of training methodology. Like high-intensity training, progressive mechanical load was devised as an attempt to apply scientific observations and principles to weight training. In a few respects, they bear some resemblance to each other: Both advocate a low volume of work, progressive resistance, and adequate recovery time. The similarities end there. Progressive mechanical load training postulates that in the case of skeletal muscles, the degree of the body's response to stress is not dependent upon the intensity of that stress. Rather, the idea is that the body responds to ever-increasing mechanical loads by building muscle tissue accordingly, and that intensity need not, and *should not*, be of the highest variety.

The reason for this is that research supporting progressive mechanical load has found that overtraining is a phenomena of the nervous system, not the muscles themselves. Inasmuch, training to or beyond failure will greatly tax the nervous system. Therefore, the recovery time required by a high-intensity workout (or a volume workout, for that matter) is due to nervous system trauma, not muscular trauma. In other words, the theory postulates that after a brutally hard high-intensity workout, within a few days the muscles have fully recovered, and essentially they must endure an inefficient waiting period while the nervous system recovers.

The research further found that muscles stimulated in a previous workout that have recovered and are in a state of adaptation (subsequent growth) can be trained during this phase, without interrupting that adaptation. Since the research found that the muscles will recover in 36-

48 hours, the training regiment prescribes a very high frequency of workouts: Each body part should be trained three times per week. In fact, the entire body should be trained in a single workout three times per week. According to the logic of the system, the moderate intensity and low volume of each exercise (one or two sets) should keep the subject from becoming overtrained. The frequency of training will allow for greatly accelerated hypertrophy—since when performed properly, every workout should result in growth.

The training regiment is divided into six-to-eight week "cycles." Progressive load is accomplished in the following manner: During each one- or two-week segment, a certain rep and weight scheme is to be used; in weeks one and two, fairly light weights and high reps are used. At week three the weights increase and the reps decrease—and so on, until in week six or eight, very high weights and very low reps are used. The idea is that the body will respond to the progression by building muscle. The subject is then to rest for one or two weeks to allow the muscles to "decondition" before starting a new cycle.

The most striking facet of progressive mechanical load training is that it attempts to refute the idea that the degree of the body's adaptive response depends upon the intensity of stress, at least in the case of skeletal muscles. A particular example used to illustrate a separate assertion of progressive mechanical load, the idea that muscles can be effectively trained during their adaptation phase, seems to (at least somewhat) contradict this. Independent of progressive mechanical load - specific research, a study was performed where the gastrocnemius muscles of animals were severed.[19] According to Haycock, the soleus muscles of these animals were therefore forced to endure a greatly increased load. Despite the greatly increased workload of the soleus, it was able to double in size and weight within days; although the muscle was working much harder and "continually loaded," it grew considerably during that time period. The study was cited as proof that muscles can grow despite being under mechanical load, and that the conventional notion of rest being required for growth is incorrect.

This example seems to have a rather large problem. First of all, exactly how much work was the soleus performing after the injury? This was not stated. It is true that in the future the animal would have to compensate for the lost gastrocnemius by greatly increased efforts of the soleus, but how much loading took place in the few days right after the injury, when the rapid growth took place? The answer is probably little to none. Animals limp when they are injured. Did they try to force these animals to walk, run, jump, etc. exactly as they had done before the injury? (And how exactly would they accomplish that?) One can imagine that this fantastic growth occurred while the animal was resting, or at least trying to avoid use of the compromised limb as much as possible—or, of course, when sleeping. Also, any load experienced by the soleus was probably proportionately far less than the load of even a moderate-intensity weightlifting workout. Mention of this example suggests that the animals, directly after the injury, placed a work load on their soleus muscles which would be equivalent to such a workout. It is difficult to imagine that this could be the case.

The idea that effective stimulation can take place while a muscle is still in a state of adaptive growth is supported by progressive mechanical load research, although to my knowledge this assertion has not achieved universal acceptance. But the most important point one might extract from the muscle-cutting experiment above is that it is inadvertently a very compelling example of the general adaptation system at work: The doubling in size of the compensating muscle is a dramatic effect. Its cause was the stress of the injury. And are many things more stressful than *completely severing a muscle*? Indeed, the degree of response matched the intensity of stress, something that progressive mechanical load training claims does not happen with regard to skeletal muscles.

This example does not disprove the progressive mechanical load training theory, but it demonstrates that its assertions regarding stress-response might be flawed or partially incorrect, and that the theory might be a bit liberal in singling out research and drawing conclusions that might support its claims. Also, there is certainly dispute about the amount of recovery time required for skeletal muscles after intense contractions, as some feel that this period could be much greater than 48 hours, especially after a high-intensity workout. But few would dispute that a range of recovery abilities exist among all weight trainers.

The idea that one can effectively stimulate growth in muscles while those muscles are still in a growth phase from a previous workout is certainly intriguing, and it will be interesting to see if other research can confirm this. It is logical to think that the lesser-intensity contractions of progressive mechanical load training will require less recovery time, but then the question becomes whether the intensity (or load actually, since progressive mechanical load training is not concerned with intensity) would be sufficient to stimulate growth. It is also logical to guess that this method will result in at least some growth (especially among new trainees) and might therefore be misconstrued as optimal or perfect (and maybe not too different from my earlier comparison of soccer building leg muscles).

HST makes some interesting claims, and unlike volume training, some specific studies have been cited in the attempt to validate it. Apart from this, progressive mechanical load training has the distinction of being part of a commercial venture (as implied by the trademarking of the HST name), since the official source of the theory also offers a line of supplements for sale that are meant to increase the effects of the training. This does not necessarily reduce the credibility of the theory or the research supporting it, but some may feel otherwise.

The effectiveness of high-intensity training has been documented, but if it turns out that the principles of progressive mechanical load training are correct, one must then deduce that high-intensity training is an approximation of progressive mechanical load training, and that better results could have been attained through its use. Along these lines, it could be concluded that high-intensity trainers use unnecessary intensity levels and unnecessarily long rest periods. It *has* been proven however, that given the right genetics and drive, the volume and high-intensity training styles can be used to build an incredibly massive physique. This has not been proven with progressive mechanical load training. But since progressive mechanical load training is a relatively new invention (circa 2000) and is thus far an extremely unpopular method, this should come as no surprise—although this is certainly not proof that it is an incorrect theory or that it does not work.

Apart from a lack of massive physiques that are the result of progressive mechanical load training, there are four primary obstacles that the method will forever have to hurdle. The first is the frequency prescribed by the method. It has been fairly well-ingrained in the minds of all but weight-training beginners that training a body part three times a week is too much. The second obstacle is the low volume prescribed by the regiment. There was much discussion earlier about the problems many have with accepting the idea that more is *not* better. Third, the method calls for moderate intensity of execution. Though good reasons are given for stopping sets short of failure, the idea that one should not work as hard as possible is counterintuitive. But of course, the low volume of work dictated by the high-intensity approach is counterintuitive as well, so hopefully we have learned to reserve judgment in such cases!

The fourth problem concerns time constraints, and is twofold: First, the method seems to mandate that for the entire six or eight week cycle, not a single workout can be missed, since an interruption might cause the body to prematurely decondition, ablating the progression that has already been established. The second part concerns the length of workouts required once the heavy weight and low-rep phase is under way. Any set of only five reps, particularly among very strong lifters, will require a fair amount of warm-up prior to execution. Suppose the subject can squat 500 pounds for five reps. He can't just hop under the bar and give it a go. It can take more than ten minutes of warm-up (or considerably longer) to reach this weight safely. After that, the subject has the remainder of a heavy full-body workout to look forward to.

A potential fifth problem, albeit one that will most likely scare few people away from the idea, is that there is hypothetically a greater risk of injury with progressive mechanical load training due to much-elevated frequency (and therefore sheer opportunity for disaster). Also, progressive mechanical load training prescribes that subjects should venture into *very* low rep ranges (five or fewer reps per set), something that high-intensity strategies generally do not suggest. In its defense, a great deal of the work performed is stopped far short of failure, and by far most of the sets are with relatively light weights. Because of this, the possibility of a muscle tear is probably low. But the threat of tendonitis, probably the most common weightlifting injury of them all, might be relatively dire due to the higher frequency of training.

Finally, there is some evidence to suggest that there might be a problem with the idea that mechanical load, and not intensity of stress, is responsible for muscular growth. If the physiques of sprinters and speed skaters are once more considered, it can be seen that the (sometimes) significant muscular growth they enjoy is purely the result of ever-increasing intensity levels, not increased load. Sprinters do not progressively increase the load of resistance in their training, only the intensity (an improvement in race time, essentially performing the same amount of work more quickly, constitutes an increase in intensity). True, they will gain some weight due to the growth of muscles, and this weight must be carried, creating a heavier load, but the overall weight gain will constitute a small extra percentage of increase—much less than the load increases prescribed by a typical progressive mechanical load training regiment. Since champion bodybuilders will always have thighs a good deal bigger than sprinters and speed skaters, one might conclude that a combination of intensity and ever-increasing mechanical load is best for inducing muscular growth.

Nevertheless, anyone who considers himself a "hard gainer" who seemingly, despite all efforts, cannot gain mass from high-intensity or any other types of training should consider giving progressive mechanical load training a try—assuming he has time for it. As mentioned above, even though it is very low-volume, one can imagine that a full-body workout will take a very long time to complete. This is especially true for advanced lifters, since it necessarily takes a while to adequately warm-up whichever muscle is being trained. For those just beginning a weight-training program, who will not have to spend a great deal of time warming up before being able to safely handle weights within the prescribed ranges, and who should not yet attempt maximum-intensity exercise anyway, progressive mechanical load training might be a good idea. In fact, it might be a fairly good way to begin a weight-training program; after completing an initial six or eight week cycle, the subject can then assess his results and then opt for a second cycle (or as many additional cycles as he sees fit) or make the transition to high-intensity training.

III

Physique

"Concentration is the secret of strength."
-Ralph Waldo Emerson

Weight training tactics

By now the importance of a theoretical foundation for a training regiment should have been established. Though taken from its original context, Emerson's comments hold true for weight training: Concentration is the secret. Mental concentration is of course critical, but the concentration of effort is of paramount importance.

The next task is to provide specific ideas about how the training regiment should be constructed, so that this concept can be properly exploited. First, here are the basics. During any training session, there should be three clearly delineated parts: Warming up, actual training (performing working or real sets) and rest.

Warm-up

The warm-up part of a workout can include two parts:

1. An initial, general warm-up, performed at the very beginning of a training session. This will often consist of light cardio work such as riding a stationary bike for 5-10 minutes or so, just enough to slightly raise the subject's heart rate. This tends to "get the blood pumping," helping to get the subject ready for the far more intense work yet to be performed; it also seems to reduce the susceptibility of the subject to moderate acute injuries such as muscle strains.
2. Weightlifting sets performed by the subject that are stopped considerably short of failure. Such sets are critical, since performing heavy, high-intensity sets without warming up first is a sure invitation to injury; also, it is very difficult to generate high intensity contractions with a "cold" muscle.

Beginners will need far fewer warm-ups than advanced subjects, since the amount of weight they will be handling will be much lower. Warm-ups should be performed by beginners nevertheless. Advanced subjects, assuming they have progressed accordingly, will need quite a few more; not only will it take longer to build up to weights that they will be using for high-intensity sets, but there is also a greater risk of injury among these people. Big, strong muscles also tear more easily. They require a greater amount of weight in order to be trained properly, naturally raising the risk level.

Also, a large number of complete-muscle-tear victims are volume trainers, and as mentioned in the *Volume and injury* section, they have a much greater predisposition to injury. I have personally known nine people that have suffered complete muscle tears. All of them are volume trainers. Obviously an anecdote does not make my conjecture on this topic a universal law, since again, Dorian Yates suffered a complete tear.

But an already worn-down muscle that is cold seems to be extremely apt to tear—since out of the nine people mentioned, three tore muscles (all biceps tears, by the way) by engaging in non-weightlifting injuries, where it should be very obvious that a deliberate warm-up did not take place. In one instance, the victim was lifting a tanning bed. In the second, the injured party suffered the tear in a fist fight. The last, quite hapless victim actually tore his right bicep while bowling!

So for each exercise, the subject ought to warm-up accordingly. As with all elements of his regiment, he must use his own discretion when devising a warm-up plan. But the warm-up period for all exercises should be fairly identical in structure: One or more very light sets, using a large number of repetitions (10 plus), each concluded well before failure is approached; one or more sets of medium weight for high reps (if more than one medium-weight set is used, then the sets should be progressively heavier); and finally, the high-intensity set itself. Below is an example of a bench-press routine for an intermediate subject:

Set 1: 135 pounds, 15 reps

Set 2: 135 pounds, 15 reps

Set 3: 185 pounds, 12 reps

Set 4: 225 pounds, 10 reps

Set 5: 255 pounds, 8 reps (this is the working set, taken to or beyond failure)

In this example, two sets are performed with 135 pounds. It is sometimes the case that more than one set is required with an initial, very light weight in order to fully warm-up before advancing to the next weight. This is certainly not a requirement, only a suggestion. Each subject should opt for whatever progression he is most comfortable. He will have to do some experimentation to figure out what is best for him.

Concerning the medium weights (sets 3 and 4), it should be noted that each set should be heavy enough to constitute a sizable progression, yet not too heavy to extend beyond what is adequate; the progression should allow the subject to comfortably transition through all the increments. Though it is best to err on the side of safety, at the same time it should be kept in mind that the subject should be keen to avoid wearing himself out by performing an excess number of warm-ups, or (as is much more often the case) by exerting too much effort—by coming too close to failure—on any of the warm-ups. The subject will not want to feel spent by the time the high-intensity set is performed. There is a slight skill to choosing the optimum number of warm-ups sets, and the weights to be used therein. This is something that comes with experience.

Many body parts should be trained with more than a single exercise, as some exercises tend to place a large amount of stress on one part of the muscle but not so much on another. The back is probably the most obvious example of this, as back workouts tend to combine a mixture of exercises intended to elicit "width" or "thickness." This being the case, a warm-up strategy that takes into account multiple exercises should be considered. In most cases, an exercise performed after the first will require less warming-up. Although I may perform as many as five warm-up sets before the very first working set of a training session, for subsequent exercises I will only perform one or two—simply because, by this point, the muscle ought to have been fully warmed-up. The warm-up sets for the later exercises will serve mainly to allow me to get a good "feel" for the exercise before using heavy weight.

Some training regiments prescribe one or more "warm-down" sets to be performed after the heaviest weights have been used; these are essentially the same as warm-up sets except that they are meant to come at the end of a number of sets (after the working sets) for a particular exercise. If warm-down sets perform any useful purpose, it is unknown to me. They are useless.

Working sets

After thoroughly warming-up, the subject ought to then perform a high-intensity set. Intensity is a relative concept, so the definition of what constitutes a high-intensity set will vary depending upon the situation. For example, in the case of some subjects, training to positive failure constitutes a degree of intensity that should be adequate to stimulate growth. In this case, the subject should continue with the set until he absolutely cannot perform another rep without assistance. Sets taken to positive failure are useful for beginners who have advanced past the initial break-in phase and intermediate lifters who are still making gains with them. Most weightlifters and bodybuilders opt to train beyond positive failure, in an attempt to produce a maximum-intensity set. Since high-intensity training is founded upon the idea that the degree of the body's response is proportional to the intensity of stress it receives, those employing it often seek to achieve the greatest levels of intensity possible. There are several tactics by which the subject can achieve this. The most popular are as follows.

Positive failure

Training to positive failure simply means that a set should be performed until the subject is no longer able to lift the weight by himself. In many cases, such sets are sufficiently intense to stimulate growth. This is particular true of beginning or intermediate subjects. In fact, it is a good idea to avoid beyond-positive-failure exercises as along as possible, the reason being that once returns begin to decrease from the positive-failure approach, there are other, more intense tactics waiting in reserve—and these more advanced methods can then be employed. If advanced tactics are used from the get-go, the subject will not have the advantage of this reserve to bump his progression back on track.

Of course, it is still possible to continually grow by using advanced tactics from the very beginning, since the subject should progress due to the action of the body's adaptation mechanism. But it seems to be more efficient to begin with less-intense methods. And make no mistake; reaching positive failure can still be extremely hard work. I've been able to achieve a great deal of strength and mass in my thighs from squatting, and I have never used any tactic besides positive failure for that exercise.

Also, when it is decided that the switch should be made from positive to beyond-positive failure due to decreasing results, the subject should make a full appraisal of his progress and efforts. Decreasing results might not necessarily be caused by insufficient intensity. In fact, a more likely culprit would be overtraining; if it turns out that the subject really is overtrained, but he opts to remedy the stagnation of his results by increasing the intensity level of his working sets, the entire effort will backfire, and things *will* get worse. That being said, any decision to attempt an increase in training intensity should not be taken lightly.

Assisted repetitions

Also known as "forced reps," the idea here is that after completing the last repetition that is possible under his own power, the subject will continue to lift the weight with the assistance of a helper or "spotter." In a normal positive failure scenario, the subject exhausts his concentric strength, thus ending the set. The benefit of the forced reps approach is that it allows the subject to exhaust his stronger eccentric strength, thus raising the intensity level of the set.

As mentioned in the "Intensity Principle" chapter in the high-intensity training section, once positive failure has been reached, the subject should slowly and deliberately lower the weight to the bottom of the range of motion of the exercise. After receiving help again in the positive portion, if the subject feels able to fully control the descent of the weight, he should attempt another such rep. Negative failure will be reached when the subject is no longer able to control the descent of the weight. At this point the set can be successfully concluded.

Over the years, I've witnessed a certain aggregate of the gym crowd using a variation of assisted reps in an attempt (I suppose) to train beyond failure, albeit often doing so in every set of a high-volume workout. When a set is performed, the actual point of positive failure ought to be unquestionably apparent to all those present: The subject, his training partner, and any observers. The technique to which I am referring actually manages to make the exact point of failure nebulous and, I guess, draws upon the same absent logic as high-volume training itself: I'm talking about a type of training you'll see amongst lifters that always train together, and always help each other lift the weight seemingly on every rep of every set. I have many times attempted to hypothesize why a training scheme like this might be a good idea, but I've yet to come up with anything.

All things being equal, muscular growth can be achieved through progressive resistance--that is, by lifting in successive workouts more weight for the same amount of repetitions, or more repetitions of the same weight, or, of course, more weight for more reps. If someone is helping you lift the weights, it doesn't take a Ph.D. in physics to deduce that the weight you are lifting is equal to the mass of the weight *minus* the force being applied by the "helper." Well, *how much is that?* Exactly how much are you lifting? The easy and correct answer is that it's impossible to tell. It is also then apparent that the actual mass of the weight being lifting is variable, because obviously the helper cannot apply exactly the same amount of force each time. And the point of failure in a set also becomes unclear, since the weight being lifted is not constant, and help is being given on every rep anyway.

The set is continued in some cases until the helper reaches "failure" before the person performing the set! For example, imagine this hapless pair blundering their way through a bench press workout. The person performing the bench presses reps away, helped by the spotter, who by action of this arrangement is performing a form of upright (or slightly bent-over) rows. As the bencher tires, the upright rows become increasing difficult, until the spotter reaches failure and must switch his posture so that he is doing something that more resembles a partial deadlift. Of course this is an extreme example, and the spotter can usually muster the strength to help the bencher complete this odd set. Of course, he's also tiring himself out a little; every possible ounce of his strength should be saved for *his* set, but this is of secondary concern.

The help-on-every-rep technique might make sense if assistance is only given during the positive portion of the movement--and the negative portion is emphasized, that is, lowered in a slow and controlled fashion. But in addition to this, such a set must be performed on rare occasions, because although this can be an effective technique, it can easily lead to overtraining. Without question, this technique should never be performed in every set of a high-volume workout. But from the fair number of weightlifters I have seen using this technique, the negative portion of any given set never seems to be slow, controlled, or unassisted. So why don't these lifters just pick a lighter weight and lift the weights themselves? Wouldn't this make a whole lot more sense? Is it inflated egos that are dictating the strategy here? And if that's the case, do these people really think that others will: 1) admire the amount of weight being lifted and 2) are at the same time willing to ignore the fact that they're not really lifting the weight? At this point I don't think I need to clarify that when I discuss forced reps, the above described training method is *not* what I'm talking about!

The main idea behind properly-executed assisted repetitions, as with all high-intensity training tactics, is that each set should be made to be more difficult, not easier. The above-described example is worthy of mention because it does not seem to have been devised with this in mind—in fact, it seems that those using it don't really have any idea what exactly they hope to achieve by using it. Probably many employ it because they have seen others doing so, and they therefore just assume that it has merit—much like volume training itself.

It should also be noted that in the case of certain exercises, forced reps can be performed alone. Single-arm dumbbell curls are one such example. The subject can use his free arm to help lift the dumbbell when positive failure has been reached. Leg press is another example. Once the subject reaches positive failure, he can assist himself during the concentric portion of each rep by pushing on his knees. Of course he should stop assisting himself during the eccentric portion, although a fair number of people seem to be forgetful or unaware of this. However, it is strongly recommended that the subject have a spotter stand nearby in case negative failure is reached and he is too momentarily weak to return the weight to the racked position.

Cheating

Although the name may seem to imply otherwise, cheating is another method whereby a set can be made more difficult and therefore more intense. The concept is relatively simple: As is the case with forced reps, a set is performed until positive failure is reached. After that, the subject will use assistance during the positive portion, and his focus will be shifted to achieving negative failure. The assistance will not come from a second-party helper, but rather from using other muscles to "cheat" the weight to the top of the movement.

Instances where cheating is most commonly used tend to be standing exercises for the upper body, and the "cheat" will often come about as a result of creating an initial vertical movement of the weight by thrusting with the legs. Once upward momentum has been established, the weight can be kept moving by the particular muscle being trained with less effort than if it were to be performed in a strict fashion. Exercises where this technique is used include barbell and dumbbell curls, front and side laterals, shrugs, standing presses, upright rows, and bent-over rows, and a few others.

Cheating is not possible with all exercises. Except for bouncing off the very bottom portion of the movement, one cannot cheat while performing squats (this technique is very dangerous for the lower back and places the subject in a very low and mechanically disadvantaged and therefore weak position anyway; you will never see experienced lifters doing this). Some will cheat on bench presses by dropping the weight from the top of the range of movement so that it crashes onto the their chests, with his ribs acting like a spring to help propel the weight as far vertical as possible before the muscles have to take over completely. Anyone that has spent much time in a gym has doubtless seen this one before. Obviously, the act of dropping the weight removes the possibility of achieving negative failure, since the weight will never be lowered in a slow, deliberate manner. And it should go without saying that one should never attempt a high-intensity set of bench presses, be they flat, incline, or decline, without a spotter on hand; a properly-performed high-intensity set of bench presses will always leave you helplessly pinned beneath the bar and in need of assistance.

Cheating with deadlifts is a virtual impossibility; also, it should be noted that cheating with any back exercise is asking for trouble, since the back tends to be prone to injury, and back training tends to involve relatively heavy weights. Because of this, it makes sense to use other high-intensity techniques to push working sets beyond positive failure. Since cheating involves the temporary manipulation of weight that is heavier than the subject can control, often achieved in a rapid, jerky fashion, the subject should use caution, and should opt to use this technique only with exercises involving relatively light weight.

Rest-pause training

Rest-pause training is another method that can be used to make a set more difficult. Once any set has been completed and failure has been achieved, the subject has reached a point where completing another rep is an impossibility. However, as soon as the set is terminated, strength begins to rapidly return to the muscle. This fact can be exploited in order to raise the intensity level of set—since with rest-pause training, the set is not over yet, and the beyond-failure portion has begun.

The idea is to wait just long enough after failure has been reached so that another, almost impossible rep can be completed. Once the adequate (albeit brief) period has elapsed, the subject should perform the rep, placing heavy emphasis on the negative portion of the movement. After another short period, another rep can be attempted, again emphasizing the eccentric contraction. By completing a set in this manner, the subject has significantly boosted its intensity level.

Mike Mentzer had a good deal of success with this technique[20]; his variation of the idea often included lifting a weight where only a single rep was possible, resting, and then lifting it again; this would be repeated a few more times. Occasionally for the last rep he would use a lower weight, since the only way to successfully perform the last rep would be with a reduced weight. I have made very good progress by performing the first portion of rest-pause sets in a more normal range, say 8-12 reps, reaching failure, and then grinding out a few rest-pause reps. The final repetition should take place when the subject feels that he will not be able to perform another rep without resting for at least a few minutes. As one might guess, rest-pause sets can be rather grueling.

One benefit of the rest-pause tactic is that it can often be performed while training alone—unlike forced reps, which requires the assistance of a spotter. There are a variety of exercises where this is possible, leg extensions and leg curls being good candidates. In fact, most machine exercises are suitable for rest-pause, since the subject need not worry about ending up trapped under the weight, as is the case with barbell-pressing type movements. This method can also be successfully applied to some free-weight upper-body movements, such as those mentioned in the Cheating section. It is important to remember that, regardless of the exercise, positive failure must truly be met before moving on to the rest-pause portion, since again, the aim here is to make the set harder, not easier.

Pre-exhaustion

The explanation of this tactic is identical to the "Pre-Exhaustion Principle" espoused by the volume training advocates: The idea is that by using this technique, one might fully isolate, and therefore most productively train, a particular muscle. This is accomplished by training that body part first with a single-joint, direct isolation exercise so that the muscle becomes fatigued, or pre-exhausted, and then immediately proceeding to a heavier, compound-type movement. The benefit is that the effectiveness of the second exercise will not be limited by the capabilities of lesser, weaker muscles.

We can use the example of a back-training workout. In this case, the subject has opted to perform barbell rows, which is a good mass-building exercise because a large number of muscle fibers are used when performed properly. But often times failure will be reached because smaller muscles (in this case, the biceps) give out before the larger, target muscle (the lats). This naturally limits the effectiveness of barbell rows as a back exercise. So the subject opts to perform a set on a lat pullover machine first, since this exercise isolates the lats and completely disinvolves the biceps. After reaching failure, he should, with as little rest as possible, proceed to the barbell rows.

While pre-exhaustion sets are technically the same as "compound sets" as described in the volume training section, the specific purpose they serve, of better isolating the target muscle, is a benefit that outweighs the primary problem of compound sets, mainly that they might reduce the intensity of the second portion of the movement. But it should be kept in mind that compounds sets constitute an arbitrary pairing of exercises, while pre-exhaustion specifies that an isolation movement should precede a compound exercise.

So it is advisable to perform a relatively low number of reps during the first phase, so that the subject is able to sustain as high a level of intensity as possible through the second portion. Mentzer advocated using a weight that will allow for six reps in the isolation movement, and this seems to be about right.[21] Reaching positive failure after six reps with a single-joint isolation movement should not leave the subject winded, and with proper motivation he should be able to attack the critical second half of the exercise with sufficient intensity.

Rest

During a training session, when not warming-up or performing working sets, the subject should be resting. The ideal amount of time that should pass from the minute one set ends and another begins will depend upon the exercise and the amount of weight being used. During the warm-up phase of lighter exercises, such as dumbbell curls, the rest period can be very brief, maybe only as long as the set itself. If the subject is particularly strong, and he is performing a heavy exercise such as squats or deadlifts, the rest period should increase; this amount of time should meet the following criteria. It should be:

1. Long enough to insure that the subject's breathing has returned to normal.
2. Long enough the subject is comfortable with commencing the next, heavier set.
3. Not so long that the subject begins to "cool down," thus increasing the chance of injury.

Even though the subject is still in the warm-up phase, some exercises will nevertheless take a toll such that a longer rest period will be required. For example, consider again the strong subject: His goal for the first exercise of a leg workout might be to squat 500 pounds for eight repetitions. His last warm-up might be with 405 pounds, where he will opt to complete ten reps. Although this is far short of the number of reps that would be required for him to achieve failure with that weight, it will still be somewhat taxing, and he will likely need to rest for a period of time longer than the length of that set before he is ready to attempt 500 with maximum intensity.

There are some people that actually time their rest periods. It seems better to subjectively determine what is best by experimenting with different lengths of rest. An optimum amount of rest insures that the subject's strength has sufficiently returned; this is especially critical right before the single maximum-intensity set, and obviously every last gram of strength must be mustered for this moment. At the same time, the rest period must not be so long that the subject has begun to cool down. What we are looking for, then, is the small window of time where both criteria are met. Again, there are no hard and fast guidelines, but through a little experimentation it shouldn't be difficult to figure out what will work best for each individual. Again, there are some that will purposely train at a quick pace in an effort to burn body fat, and achieve a "hard" or "toned" look. The explanation of the Specificity Principle (p. 36) describes the problems with this approach.

Time under tension

In recent years it has been popular to talk about "time under tension" for weightlifting exercises, the idea being that the amount of time a muscle is placed under stress (the total length of a set) is more important than the actual number of repetitions being performed. It has been further postulated that the optimum amount of time under tension should depend upon the type of muscle fibers the subject seeks to stimulate. There are three types of such fibers: Fast twitch, slow twitch, and intermediate/mixed fiber type.

Individuals vary as to the ratio of such fibers in their composition. Beyond this, certain muscles tend to have a greater concentration of one or the other. For example, triceps tend to be composed predominately fast-twitch fibers. This makes sense, since the purpose of the triceps is to push things away. It's easy to imagine that this can be most useful if we are able to push things away very quickly (the specialty of the fast-twitch fiber) and with a good deal of force. With this in mind, it might help to consider the idea of prehistoric man. Being able to quickly push something or someone away quickly might mean the difference between eating and going hungry, or even between life and death.

In contrast to this, the biceps have a higher concentration of slow-twitch fibers. Again, this is understandable, since the purpose of the biceps is to supinate the hand and lift objects higher or closer to the body. It can be imagined that there would be much less need to do this in a quick, violent fashion than with the "pushing away" scenario suggested above. Biceps are useful for carrying things (ask any mother with a six-month old baby how her biceps feel from carrying the infant), and are able to do so for extended periods.

It has therefore been suggested that different muscles or fiber types should be subject to different amounts of time under tension. 30-50 seconds is generally prescribed for predominantly fast-twitch fiber muscles, with 90-120 seconds for slow-twitch, and 50-80 seconds for the intermediate types. While these numbers should be kept in mind, it is not advisable to construct sets around a stop-watch. In fact, the most practical point to be taken from the consideration of different fiber types is that it is generally best to train the lower body (which tends to have, in general, a large number of slow-twitch fibers) with higher reps than the upper.

After all, the best way to insure progression in the gym is by keeping track of the weight and amount of repetitions used for all exercises. A rep range of 6-12 for upper-body and 8-20 (and even higher) for lower body exercises, when performed slowly and deliberately, tend to allow for a time under tension that is similar to the guidelines specified above. In other words, it's good to be aware of the concept of time under tension, but the concept of progression, as measured by the weights the subject is using and repetitions he is performing, should be considered more important.

Since all muscles have both slow- and fast-twitch fibers, to insure that the maximum number of fibers become subject to stimulation, it is not beyond the bounds of reason to allow for two high-intensity sets per exercise—one emphasizing higher reps and time under tension, the other of a lower variety. Anyone attempting this approach should be keen to note the onset of any symptoms of overtraining, however. Such a routine can still be considered low-volume, but of course it is falls outside the guidelines of strict Mentzerian HIT. It is certainly not volume training, however.

Such an approach might be appropriate for beginning or intermediate lifters who are not yet using the type of weights that, when used with high-intensity techniques, require significant recuperation, as is the case with advanced high-intensity lifters. Also, if it is decided that the subject should employ two working sets per exercise, fewer overall exercises should be used. For example, instead of a chest workout employing one working set each of incline, flat, and decline presses, the subject might use two sets each of inclines and declines; the heavier sets should use 6-8 reps, with the lighter sets adjusted so that 12-15 (or even higher) reps are used. But there is never a good reason to perform more than two working sets per exercise.

Staggered progression

It can sometimes be physically and psychologically daunting to achieve progression, in successive training sessions for a particular body part, with the number of repetitions performed with a certain weight, or by lifting more weight for equal number of reps. For example, consider the former model of progression: Say a subject is able to perform eight reps with 275 pounds in the bench press. In the next chest workout, he has chosen to use 275 once more for his working set. If he is progressing properly, then he should be able to get nine or more this time around. However, failure to top his previous best effort with that weight—failing to make progress with the bench press—will potentially signal an even greater failure, since theoretically his entire progression will have come to a halt. There can be many causes for this, the most likely of which being overtraining.

But let's assume that he is not overtraining. There is a vast array of variables in the equation, and one should not underestimate the psychological angle. At least subconsciously the subject knows that failure to progress in this one instance could be symptomatic of a general foundering of the effort—even if there is no rational basis for the fear, and the subject is adhering to a sound strategy and training hard. Something as innocuous as a sudden, ill-timed intrusive thought can throw off one's concentration, causing the execution of a set to falter. In the case of high-intensity training, there is little room for such lapses in concentration. The chapter on the "zone" state of mind (in the *Intangibles* section) will attempt to shed some light on the mechanism of concentration. But sometimes a hidden (or not-so-hidden) fear of failure can derail the execution of set. After all, if our overall progression is a state dependent upon the progression of specific increases in strength, then a certain amount of self-induced psychological pressure exists to keep things moving forward.

This is an area where those with a fierce competitive spirit will excel. Indeed, one should learn to relish the opportunity to rise to the occasion, *to show what he is made of,* if he is to be most successful. In *The Face of Battle,* historian John Keegan noted that perhaps the most important attribute an army can have is its desire to win. This is true for bodybuilding as well. Of course, desire alone will not lead to victory. It is critical to have a good strategy, and it's helpful to employ good tactics. I have found staggered progression to be one such tactic.

Apart from mastering the ability to concentrate mentally, which should translate into the ability to muster a supremely concentrated effort, a simple technique can be useful for surmounting the potential psychological obstacle of progression. Essentially, one should endeavor to progress with more than one weight. Inasmuch, a combination of three weights seems to work well, so I will use this example to illustrate the method. In any given workout, one of the three weights will be used for the single working set for a particular exercise.

The above-mentioned subject is currently benching 275 pounds for eight reps, which he did in his last chest-training session. So for the following workout, he can choose one of two other weights, say 260 or 290 (these are given as examples only; the exact poundages should be determined at the discretion of the subject). For this session he'll be training with 260. His goal will be to break his record with that weight. The last time he trained to failure with 260 he was able to get 12 reps, so this time he's attempting to get 14. The session after that, he will be using 290. His previous best was five, so now he's after at least six. Finally, after the sessions with 260 and 290 he will return to train with 275, attempting to top his previous best with that weight. And once adequate progression is established with all weights, the subject can drop the lowest weight from the regiment, and add a new highest weight (maybe 305 this time around). Essentially the subject will be "leap-frogging" his target training weights. Here is a summary of the progression:

Workout 1: 275x8

Workout 2: 260x14

Workout 3: 290x6

Workout 4: 275x10

Workout 5: 265x14

Workout 6: 290x7

...and so forth.

Although intensity levels are theoretically rising with every workout, there is measurable progression between sessions 1 and 4, 2 and 5, and 3 and 6. In training session 5, the weight was raised because the rep range (14+) was starting to get too high.

I have personally found this method to be psychologically beneficial. Of course, a method that allows for a superior psychological state and therefore improved performance is necessarily physically beneficial as well. As far as physical benefit independent of any psychological propping, it is of course possible to increase intensity levels (and therefore create new levels of physiological impression, or stimulation, given to the muscle during the training session), from one session to the very next even though different weights and rep ranges are being used. The benefit of this ever-increasing intensity will be realized when the subject continues to break records with all the target weights. The staggering of weights also helps to reduce the familiarity of the situation slightly, which by itself can help boost motivation. I hope not to imply that the moving around of target weights will alleviate boredom, because anyone finding their workouts to be boring should probably look for another pastime!

My most notable success with this tactic was when I used it for my squatting routine. I would use as many as five target weights, and would often make very steady progress in the amount of reps I was able to perform for each weight—often for periods of greater than six months. The result was a significant gain in mass.

Beginning routines

The purpose of a beginning routine should be acclimation to weightlifting. Attempting to jump right in and perform a high-intensity workout from day one will result in chronic, even temporarily disabling muscle soreness. Apart from that, high-intensity techniques are not needed yet. The muscles will begin to grow using less intense techniques, and as pointed out in the section on positive failure, to use high-intensity methods from the start will deny the subject a strategic reserve of tactics that will help boost his progress when they are really needed. But in very early stages, they are not needed, and they are excessive.

The first week or two of training should be composed mainly of training with light weights, to get the subject's muscles accustomed to weight-training; this will also provide a rough gauge of what amount of weight he should be using for all of the exercises. Since the beginning weightlifter will spend a very small amount of time training each body part, and he will not be training to failure, it is advisable to train the entire body in each session. It is further recommended that he use no more than two exercises per body part.

If the subject is training at a large gym, such as many of the Gold's Gyms, the sheer number of machines and free weights might seem bewildering. But for any single regiment, regardless of the experience level of the subject, a very small percentage of the total number of machines and free weight stations will be used. This being the case, it is natural for the beginner to feel that he is "missing out" by not using most of the machines at his disposal. As a beginner, I recall feeling this way. However, this worry can be quelled once it is realized that among the large variety of machines and free-weight exercises, there is a great deal of redundancy of effect. One back machine, for example, might work the back in a nearly identical manner to another machine, despite the difference in appearance between the two.

For the advanced lifter, the choice between two machines (or free-weight exercises) that have only subtle differences primarily becomes a matter of personal preference. For example, my choice to use certain machines sometimes boils down to how much total resistance is available on the weight stack, since sometimes my strength exceeds that total weight available on others. Often the determination about which machine to use can be made during the warm-up phase of a workout, so that the subject need not use a different exercise every workout until he reaches a decision. As pointed out previously, frequent exercise changes can undermine the subject's progress, since using the exact same exercise in subsequent workouts is the only objective way to insure that the principle of progression is applied properly.

So it is perfectly acceptable, advisable even, for the subject to try a few different machines that have a similar purpose as he warms up. Again, we will use the example of back machines. The great majority fall into two categories: Those involving a "pull down," and those involving a "rowing" type of movement. Pull downs tend to emphasize involvement of the latisimus dorsi muscles (lats), and are thus categorized as "width" movements, and rows tend to include all muscles of the back, including the spinal erectors, and are thus often thought of as thickness-producing. (There is a third category, that of pullovers; these are able to directly isolate the lat muscles because the resistance of the machine is applied by the upper arms to pads on the machine, thus disinvolving the arm muscles).

There is a very wide array of machines available for both types of movements, but again, personal preference should dictate which ones should be used. Each machine will have its own unique geometry, and the subject will find that one particular machine might suit his physical structure better than others. The identity principle makes clear the fact that we all share a uniform physiology, but our dimensions are all unique, so this is indeed one instance where we are all different. The subject will know which machine is best by determining which machine seems to place the most direct stress on the target muscles. For instance, with some back machines, I am able to feel the back muscles working better than with others, which might seem to overly involve the biceps or shoulders.

It also critical to learn proper form; this will enable the subject to enjoy the optimal effect of any given exercise, and will help steer him clear of injury. This is particularly true of squats, which are performed in a wrong and dangerous fashion more often that not. Unless you are absolutely sure that your form is perfect on all exercises, it might be worthwhile to hire a personal trainer to help you with the finer points.

That being said, the initial period should consist of visiting the gym three times per week, training the entire body in each session. The weights should be kept light, and the amount of effort exerted should not be great. At the same time, however, the subject should pay attention the amount of weight that he can comfortably lift, so that later on, when the intensity levels are notched up, he will have a rough idea about how heavy he should be training. The following is an example of such an introductory workout, with a few light sets performed for each:

Leg press or squats

Smith machine bench press

Wide-grip pulldowns

Machine rows

Machine shoulder presses

Side laterals

Barbell curls

Cable triceps pushdowns

Leg curls

Donkey calf raises

Incline bench sit-ups

Of course, there are a large number of exercises that can be substituted for the above, and by no means should this be considered a set-in-stone list. For example, dumbbell curls can be substituted for barbell curls; T-bar rows can be substituted for machine rows, and so forth. Once again, since the aim here is acclimation, the subject should not attempt to put forth a great deal of effort. If he does, he will find himself pretty worn out by the end of the workout—and he definitely doesn't want to find himself in an overtrained state after less than two weeks in the gym!

Intermediate routines

For our purposes, an "intermediate" routine will be one that employs to-failure training; later advanced routines will use beyond-failure methods. As far as what defines an intermediate bodybuilder or weightlifter, that will depend upon his level of development and/or strength. There is no objective definition for this, although one might expect to endure up to a few years of steady progress before being considered "advanced." At the same time, it is reasonable (and common) for a subject with an intermediate physique to have graduated to an advanced training routine, depending upon his progression.

After the initial break-in period, the subject can opt for one of two distinct paths: Either an intermediate, high-intensity precursory regiment, or progressive mechanical load training. The former will normally consist of a three- or four-day split, with two sets per exercise taken to failure. Here are two examples (warm-up sets are not specified, as it should be left to the discretion of the subject as to how much warming-up he should do per what is described in the Warm-Up section) of such a regiment. Each working set should be taken to positive failure, but not beyond:

Routine 1

Day 1: Chest, shoulders, and triceps

Incline press	x2
Decline or bench press	x2
Military press	x2
Side Laterals	x2
Lying triceps extensions	x2

Day 2: Back, biceps, and abs

Wide-grip pulldowns	x2
Barbell rows	x2
Barbell curls	x2
Hanging leg raises	x2

Day 3: Legs

Squats or leg press	x2
Leg extensions	x2
Lying leg curls	x2
Donkey calf raises	x2

Day 4: Rest

Routine 2

Day 1: Chest and triceps

Incline press	x2
Decline or bench press	x2
Close-grip bench press	x2
Lying triceps extensions	x2

Day 2: Back, biceps, and abs

Wide-grip pulldowns	x2
Barbell rows	x2
Low pulley rows	x2
Barbell curls	x2
Hanging leg raises	x2

Day 3: Thighs and calves

Squats or leg press	x2
Leg extensions	x2
Thigh adductors	x2
Donkey calf raises	x2

Day 4: Shoulders and hamstrings

Military press	x2
Side Laterals	x2
Rear-delt lateral raises	x2
Shrugs	x2
Lying leg curls	x2

Day 5: Rest

Again, many of the exercises specified can be interchanged with others. The second example is a bit more advanced, and the addition of an extra day allows for greater specialization of exercises: For example, thighs and hamstrings as well as chest and shoulders have been separated, and extra exercises have been added for some body parts.

Construction of an individual regiment ought to reflect the priorities of the subject; for example, if his thigh development lags behind the rest of his physique, he might consider training that body part following a day of rest, since his energy levels will be higher, and he can naturally devote more effort to that day of training. In another example, an individual that has proportionately greater gluteus development might elect to remove regular squats from his program, since apart from being the most effective quadriceps exercise, they are even more effective for glute development; he might use leg presses or front squats instead, since these involve the glutes to a lesser degree.

It is also perfectly acceptable (and actually, a very good idea) in the case of a four-day split to include two rest days, such that the regiment can be described as two-on, one-off, two-on, one-off. In the second example above, the first day of rest would come after the back/biceps/abs day. Overtraining is rampant among intermediate lifters, so one must always take measure of his progress and pay close attention to his body's response above and beyond the simple progression of weights and repetitions; in particular, he should look for any signs of overtraining. The principle of frequency states that an individual absolutely *must* allow for enough time to recover from a workout, so this point should be taken seriously.

Intermediate routines must also employ workouts of sufficient intensity. In this stage of training, taking each set to positive failure should provide adequate intensity of stress, thereby stimulating growth. But remember to train hard! Training with a high level of motivation will translate into greater output, more reps, and therefore more and faster growth. As mentioned previously, with a well-executed workout plan, progression should take care of itself, but this is another factor that must be kept in mind: Weights and repetitions must be increased regularly to insure progression of growth.

The idea of performing two sets to failure for each exercise in the above examples presents a conflict with the strict single-set high-intensity formula. However, for sub-advanced routines, the benefits might outweigh any possible detriment. There appear to be a few advantages: As mentioned in the Time Under Tension chapter, all muscles have both fast-and slow-twitch fibers, and evidence suggests that different amounts of time under tension (or for all intents and purposes, repetition ranges) can be more beneficial for one or the other. This being the case, one working set each of lower (6-8) and higher (10-15) reps might be an effective way to exploit this. Whereas in the case of advanced lifters, where the addition of just one more set per exercise might be markedly detrimental due to the amount of weight being lifted and intensity generated (with extra recovery therefore being required), less-advanced subjects are less apt to make significant inroads into their recovery process by doing so. In short, for intermediate lifters, the danger of "overdoing it" by employing a second set is not great.

There is also the psychological factor to consider. Many sub-advanced lifters just cannot be satisfied with performing a single high-intensity set, even if they have complete trust in the logic of the method.

At one time I fell into this category, so before fully committing to the single-set approach, for most exercises I would perform two sets. (This should still be considered low-volume training). Apart from psychological satisfaction with the workload in general, there is specific satisfaction to be gained from, in essence, having two opportunities to create maximum effort. Let's face it; being able to produce maximum intensity at will is not easy, and for most, it is a skill to be learned. And for most people (since the majority will fall into the sub-advanced category), performing a second set will at worst be only slightly detrimental—and it is certainly a far better alternative to following a volume training regiment, which depending upon the individual and the program, can be highly counterproductive and inefficient. But there is never a good reason to do more than two working sets per exercise.

Progressive mechanical load training regiment

Progressive mechanical load training (or "Hypertrophy-Specific Training") is fairly new and somewhat controversial, but upon becoming aware of it I realized that it might make for a good early-stage routine— and if it produces satisfactory results among those opting to give it a try, I heartily encourage continuing with it, since it is theoretically useful for intermediates and advanced lifters as well. One thing that makes this type of training unique is that it requires the strict devotion by the subject to a six- or eight-week "cycle." With other types of training, an occasional interruption of a few days or even a week is not a big deal (and most people will actually benefit from it), but with progressive mechanical load training, any such intermission can cause an entire month or two of effort to be lost.

The reason for this (as mentioned in the progressive mechanical load training section, pages 83-88) is that the foundation of the strategy is the idea that muscles grow as a result of adapting to ever-increasing mechanical loads. Week after week the weights get progressively heavier, culminating in the final two weeks, which feature the use of very heavy weights.

Unlike the case where the subject will be transitioning into a pre-HIT routine, with progressive mechanical load training, he absolutely must establish his exact strength levels for certain rep ranges for all exercises. For example, he must know the maximum amount of weight he can lift for 5, 10, and 15 reps for all exercises. The reason for this is that the subject can then build up to using (during the course of a one- or two-week sub-cycle) that weight, thus subjecting the muscle to increasing mechanical load. Accordingly, a beginner will need extra time in the gym to establish what these poundages will be.

Once this has been done, he can begin the training. As mentioned previously, the entire body ought to be trained three times per week. The following is an example of a collection of exercises that will work the entire body.

Leg press or squats

Leg curls

Bench press

Wide-grip pulldowns

Machine rows

Machine shoulder presses

Side laterals

Barbell curls

Cable triceps pushdowns

Donkey calf raises

Incline bench sit-ups

When selecting exercises, it has been recommended that whenever possible, one should select compound exercises over isolation types, since compound movements place a greater mechanical load on the muscles. After warming up, the subject should perform one or two working sets per exercise. Keep in mind that progressive mechanical load training working sets are different from HIT working sets, in that except where indicated, these sets are *not* taken to failure.

Weeks one and two will concentrate on low repetition ranges (15). Although these six workouts will use 15 reps for all sets, the amount of weight will increase with each workout. For example, suppose the subject can bench 155 pounds for 15 reps maximum; in the first training session (Monday of week one), he might use only 105 pounds, and he will stop at 15 reps. Although he should clearly have the ability to lift a great many more repetitions, he should stop there nevertheless. The idea here is not to drain the body, and certainly not to reach failure—only to establish a mechanical load that will be topped a couple of days later. Apart from that, the combination of the high frequency required by progressive mechanical load training and high intensity levels will quickly cause the subject to overtrain.

So the entire two-week sub-cycle for bench press portion of the workout might look like the following:

Week one

Monday	105x15
Wednesday	115x15
Friday	125x15

Week two

Monday	135 x15
Wednesday	145x15
Friday	155x15

Weeks three and four will be similar, expect with heavier weights and lower reps. Again, here is a hypothetical bench press example:

Week three

Monday	125x10
Wednesday	135x10
Friday	145x10

Week four

Monday	155x10
Wednesday	165x10
Friday	175x10

Weeks five and six are similar, except that five reps should be used instead of ten, with an appropriate adjustment of poundages. If, at that point, the subject opts to extend the entire cycle another two weeks, he can repeat what was performed in weeks five and six (although theoretically he could raise the poundages slightly, as by this point his strength might have increased, and the upward bump with the weights will translate into greater mechanical load). It is also possible to decrease rep ranges every week, instead of every two weeks. An example of such a six-week cycle might include weeks featuring the following reps: 15, 12, 10, 8, 6, 4. The important thing is that for each repetition specified for a particular week, the weights should keep increasing—and that each week should entail a lower rep scheme than the week that preceded it.

At the completion of the cycle, the subject should rest for at least a week. Progressive mechanical load training theory refers to this period as "strategic deconditioning." This period of rest will allow the body to recover in a general sense from the prior regiment, but it is further supposed that the muscles themselves will reset their reference point from the campaign of ever-increasing mechanical load—which, after all, is the purpose of the strategy. Theoretically, after a suitable period of deconditioning has elapsed, the subject will be recharged, and the muscles will be ready for a new progression of loading. And if all went according to plan, the subject should be stronger and bigger.

Using hypertrophy-specific training as a beginning-to-intermediate option has been recommended for three main reasons:

1. Some people claim to get good results from it.
2. Unlike many training systems, it has a theoretical foundation.
3. It theoretically fits the criteria for an early-stage routine, due to the acclimation and gradually-increasing difficulty which are central to the strategy.

Points one and two suggest that subsequent and indefinite cycles of progressive mechanical load training might be used to good effect—and that it might have value as an advanced program. As pointed out in the discussion of progressive mechanical load training theory, there might be some problems with its theoretical foundation, but the idea of increased mechanical load as the primary mechanism for hypertrophy is enticing. Apart from that, it does not share the potential (and very often) destructive identity of volume training, iterations of which regularly prescribe a wildly excessive workload. Progressive mechanical load training recommends an extremely high frequency of work, but low volume and variable (albeit often only moderate) intensity. For this reason it meets the third criteria listed above.

Although the subject needs to establish the limitations of his strength beforehand, the regiment prescribes gradually increasing levels of mechanical load, the side-effect being that intensity levels will creep upwards as well. By the time the first cycle is completed, he will be ready to switch to a high-intensity regiment or initiate another progressive mechanical load training cycle. He might ultimately find himself opting to pursue high-intensity training, since apart from its proven effectiveness, it is much more time-efficient. For an advanced subject with superior strength levels, the allotment of time for warm-up alone for a full-body training session is certain to be quite lengthy.

So a subject graduating from hypertrophy-specific to high-intensity training should be fairly comfortable with elevating the intensity levels of his sets as need be, since as mentioned, a necessary by-product of increased load is increased intensity. Although a subject embarking on a high-intensity program need not submit to the lengthy workouts or rigid scheduling requirements of progressive mechanical load training, he absolutely must become accustomed to generating intensity, on-demand.

If forced to make a choice, I would recommend the more conventional pre-HIT routine for those starting out with weight-training over progressive mechanical load training, for the following reasons:

1. Although some claim to have success with progressive mechanical load training (and granted, the idea is more or less theoretically sound), it can still be considered experimental.
2. The more conventional pre-HIT approach has been proven to be effective.
3. Progressive mechanical load training has very stringent time and scheduling requirements; it seems that its effectiveness will drop off markedly if any workouts are missed, postponed, or abbreviated; the pre-HIT routines are more forgiving in this regard.

Advanced routines

Advanced routines are for lifters who have mastered the ability to generate the highest levels of intensity, on-demand, and who are training with poundages that are likely to induce overtraining or at least impinge upon the subject's progress if more than a single set per exercise is performed. Although this will vary depending upon the individual, it should be assumed that, under normal circumstances, anyone with more than a year of training under his belt stands to do more harm than good by performing more than a single high-intensity set per exercise. Advanced routines also tend to feature the beyond-failure techniques listed on pages 95-100, which will of course increase the effectiveness of a workout (or the detriment thereof, should an excessive workload be performed).

The primary features of advance routines are maximum intensity, brevity, and infrequency. Since these routines for the most part will include a single working set for each exercise, the two most critical variables then become 1) the number of exercises per body part, and 2) the number of rest days between each training session. It is up to the subject what the answer will be for each—although high-intensity theory itself makes clear the idea that an excessive effort, be it through too many total sets or too little rest (or both) should be considered counterproductive or in the worst of cases, totally destructive.

Many high-intensity trained bodybuilders and weightlifters perform a number of exercises per body part such that they are satisfied that the muscle has been fully stimulated, from all angles. For example, regardless of training strategy, nearly all chest workouts feature exercises that place emphasis on the upper pecs (such as incline presses or flyes) as well as the lower pecs (declines). High-intensity workouts are no exception; this being the case, I have found that a single set each of machine incline and decline presses provides a very effective overall chest workout. Other advanced lifters will add a set of flyes (cable crossovers being a popular iteration), bumping the total number of sets to three. Many find this routine to be wildly understated, but again, this is the nature of the beast in a universe of physique culture that remains shackled to the more-is-better "logic." And remember, apart from its effectiveness, this approach is far safer than the standard volume approach.

The human back is fairly complex in its arrangement and function, so understandably back workouts tend to feature a relatively large number of exercises. Back workouts will often include a lower-back exercise, such as deadlifts or hyperextensions; pullovers to isolate the lats; pulldowns or chins as a compound lat exercise, and a rowing movement for the lats and spinal erectors. This being the case, four or five exercises for the back is a reasonable work load. There are a vast number of different back exercises and machines; many stimulate the back muscles in only a slightly different manner, so in essence, there is a great deal of redundancy among them. This should be kept in mind when formulating a training regiment, since it's important to avoid redundant efforts.

Smaller muscles are easier to fully stimulate. It's possible to get an effective bicep workout by performing only barbell curls, although many (myself included) opt to employ different exercises for the upper and lower portions of the muscle. Likewise, deltoids can be optimally trained by performing a single exercise each for the front, side, and rear heads of the muscle.

The chapter on the Frequency Principle (pages 33-35) addresses the issue of how often one should train each body part. For the advanced lifter taking each working set beyond failure, at least four days should elapse before training any body part again (as in the case of a three-on, one-off split). In most cases, there should be a good deal more rest. Nowadays many bodybuilders use a once-a-week regiment. This should be considered adequate for almost all advanced lifters, and I used this strategy for several years with very good results.

The following is an example of an advanced routine. For each exercise, a single set should be taken to or beyond failure:

Day 1: Quadriceps and Calves

Squats

Leg extensions

Thigh adductors

Donkey calve raises

Day 2: Chest, triceps, and abs

Incline press

Decline press

Lying triceps extensions

Triceps pushdowns

Hanging leg raises

Machine crunches

Day 3: Back and biceps

Machine pullovers

Wide-grip pulldowns

Barbell rows

Hyperextensions

Concentration curls

Preacher curls

Day 4: Rest

Day 5: Hamstrings, glutes, and forearms

Lying leg curls
Seated leg curls
Machine glute kick-backs
Wrist curls

Day 6: Shoulders

Military press
Machine side laterals
Bent-over dumbbell laterals
Dumbell shrugs

Day 7: Rest

This is only an example. There are unlimited combinations of body parts per session, specific exercises, and number and frequency of rest days that can make an effective system.

Single set vs. fiber-specific training

It was earlier mentioned that at least theoretically, different rep ranges should affect different muscle fiber types differently: Higher reps are more effective for slow-twitch fibers, and lower reps are more effective for fast-twitch types. Whereas two working sets per exercise can be a reasonable recommendation for beginning-to-intermediate routines—with a higher and lower repetition range for each, two working sets for an advanced subject can very often be less effective, due to the increased recovery demands and, of course, the fact that there is not a cumulative benefit of growth stimulation from performing additional sets.

A potential problem with performing a single set is that the muscle being trained by a certain exercise will of course be limited to a specific rep range—so theoretically not all fibers will receive optimum stimulation. This is a theoretical problem with a theoretical solution. It is very common to train each body part with more than a single exercise, to insure that all fibers in that muscle have been adequately stimulated. For any single body part, there is going to be a redundancy of effect when more than one exercise is used. For example, for biceps, concentration curls are used to place maximum stress on the upper portion of that muscle, and preacher curls are used to insure proper stimulation of the lower region. Nevertheless, both exercises are going to place stress on some of the same fibers, and possibly on *all* of the same fibers.

This being the case, it might be a good idea to use higher reps for one movement, and lower reps for the other—and that this rep scheme should be alternated: One workout should feature higher reps for preacher curls and lower reps for concentration curls; the next should feature lower reps for preacher curls and higher reps for concentration curls. Such an alternating arrangement of weights and sets could easily be made to be consistent with the idea of staggered progression (p. 104).

However, as mentioned, the problem of needing to address both fiber types but limiting each exercise to one set is theoretical. There have been many bodybuilders that have made excellent gains using single-set high-intensity training while not deviating far from a particular repetition range, six or eight reps being an example. And again, performing more than two working sets per exercise should always be considered detrimental. Performing a third set with the idea that the medium-twitch fibers need to be specifically addresses is never a good idea, either. These fibers should have received sufficient stimulation by the first two sets. The third set will be excessive and counterproductive.

Types of exercises

There are two primary types of weightlifting exercises:

1. Compound (also known as "basic") exercises. These are movements that feature the use of more than one joint. These are considered to be essential for building mass, since they stimulate the greatest number of muscle fibers.
2. Isolation exercises. These are movements that feature the use of only a single joint. They are considered to be less effective for building mass, but as the name implies, they are useful for isolating and therefore fully stimulating any muscle.

An effective mass-building routine must be constructed around compound exercises. It's very common to see lifters who have built a slight amount of muscle performing endless sets of isolation exercises such as cable crossovers. Apart from the problems of the high-volume approach which have been discussed at great length, somehow the idea has been instilled in a large number of people that exercises like this are the key to growth. They are not. Cable crossovers can sometimes be useful because they allow the pectoral muscles to fully contract while still under the load of weight—and this can translate to slightly improved inner-chest development—but they are unable to offer a degree of stimulation remotely approaching what can be achieved through the premier compound chest movement, bench presses. So for the purpose of training for mass, isolation movements should never be performed when a superior compound movement is available. It is little wonder that most of the cable crossover fanatics have little muscle to speak of.

However, it should be noted that although some muscles benefit a good deal from compound movements, their development is often primarily the result of isolation exercises. Hamstrings are a good example. Squats, leg presses, and deadlifts—all compound movements—stress the hamstrings considerably, but for the majority of people the most effective exercise for this muscle is lying leg curls. Biceps and calves also fall into this category, but muscles that grow more readily from isolation movements are the exception rather than the rule.

Isolation movements have their place, to be sure, and should always play some part in a mass-building regiment—since they allow for direct and concentrated stimulation of body parts like those listed above. As mentioned previously, they can be invaluable for some who are able to extract great benefit from the pre-exhaustion tactic. But basic exercises are the foundation of mass-building, and should be prioritized accordingly.

Free weights vs. machines

Apart from the two primary categories listed above, there are two sub-types of exercises: Free weights and machines. There are compound and isolation movements for both types. There are benefits and disadvantages to both.

A popular notion is that free weights are superior for building mass. This idea probably originated back before the advent of the exercise machine revolution, when most gyms had only a few machines, and only a small number had any of respectable design. Apart from dubious conception, many machines were designed for isolation-type movements (which tend to be inferior for mass-building) and/or did not have much weight available on the pin-loaded stack—and both of these points would help sway the opinion that machines are universally inferior. There are now high-quality machines that are able to emulate every movement that can be performed with free weights. Apart from this, there are movements that can *only* be optimally performed on machines. I will once more use the example of leg curls to illustrate this point. One can certainly train the hamstrings by using free weights only, but not to full effect; indeed, leg curls are necessary for optimal hamstring development.

Machines also allow subjects to train alone. Many people, myself included, do not use training partners. Training to or beyond failure with many exercises is an impossibility when alone. Spend enough time in a gym and eventually you will see someone trapped beneath a barbell on the bench press; he will be training alone and attempting one last rep in the hope of reaching positive failure. The problem is that he will have apparently unknowingly reached positive failure on his last rep. A much better alternative would have been to use a version of machine presses, or barbell presses on a Smith machine. With the latter, even when trapped, the victim can rack the weight on the nearest notch and slide out from under it.

In contrast, a variety of beyond-failure techniques can be used when training alone on machines. For bench presses, a set can be ended with a slow negative, and terminated as described above. Rest-pause sets can also be readily performed on machines.

One problem with machines is that they confine the subject to a restricted, pre-set motion. This is another problem that has been remedied to a large extent by improved design of newer models. Machines now are highly adjustable and in some cases offer additional joints which allow a second plane of movement (such as back machines that allow the handles to be moved inward or outward in addition to the primary resistance of the forward-and-back motion). Evidence suggests that the restricted motion of machines is not necessarily or significantly detrimental.

The greatest problem with machines, one that will never be fully remedied no matter how ingenious the design, is that machines have some degree of friction in their range of motion—a problem nonexistent with free weights (other than the friction of air as the weight travels through it; but the effects of aerodynamics on weightlifting is so miniscule that it is not worthy of consideration!). The problem is this: When friction exists in a machine, it will always require more force to lift the weight than to lower it. To illustrate this point, imagine using a *very* poorly-lubricated machine, in this case a flat bench press unit. Lifting the weight might take a great deal of effort. Part of the resistance will come from the weight being lifted, and part of it will come from the friction of the machine. The fact that part of the resistance is a result of friction, at least in the positive portion of the movement, is immaterial. Resistance is resistance.

However, once the positive portion of the movement has been completed, the problem caused by friction increases markedly. The top of the movement, the static contraction, will be easier than it should be. The friction will help hold the weight at the top of the movement. (In the case of very poorly-cared for equipment, an un-lubricated machine might even actually stay stuck at the top of the range of movement! I have actually attempted to use machines that were this bad, many years ago.) The negative portion of the exercise will be even easier, since friction will help slow the descent of the weight.

This is the opposite of what is ideal. The negative portion of a movement should be at least as (or more) difficult than the positive. The previous description of the benefits of positive and negative failure as well as assisted repetitions makes clear this point. Even the most efficiently-designed, well-lubricated machines have some friction, which will naturally decrease their effectiveness. In this regard, free weights can be thought of as superior.

One often-cited reason for the supposed universal superiority of free weights is that the unrestricted path of travel of the weight will necessarily cause the involvement of additional muscles which will be forced to exert effort to balance the weight. For example, with machine bench presses, the subject need only be concerned with lifting the weight and lowering it in the single plane of the movement. With free weight bench presses, the subject must lift and lower the weight, but he must also balance the weight so that the barbell does not fall off to one side. It is thought that the act of balancing will result in greater muscular growth. This is incorrect. The "balancing" muscles are being subjected to stress, but this stress in no way approaches the level of intensity required to stimulate those muscles to grow. It is a far better idea to train the balancing muscles using direct, intense exercise. Furthermore, the energy spent balancing the weight is just that: Energy spent. The subject is burning a few extra calories by balancing the weight, but he is also imposing upon himself some unproductive energy expenditure. So the act of balancing the weight, commonly thought to be beneficial, is actually slightly counterproductive.

One advantage with many machines is that, unlike many free weight exercises, they allow for there to be high levels of resistance throughout the full range of motion. An example of this would be the difference in resistance available for free weight and machine preacher curls. In free weight preacher curls, at the top of the range of motion, the forearms are more or less perpendicular to the floor. There is little or no resistance in this position, with the weight is mainly just being balanced. Obviously there is little to be gained from the top portion of the range of motion of this exercise. In contrast, machine preacher curls subject the biceps to even resistance throughout the range of motion, including the top portion.

Likewise, cable crossovers provide full resistance throughout the range of motion—unlike pressing movements, where there will be less resistance at the top portion of the movement due to the mechanical considerations; since the top of a bench press involves only the straightening of an almost-straight arm, the mechanical advantages are rather large. It is for this reason that *very* heavy weights can be handled in the very top portion of the range of motion of pressing-style movements. However, this advantage with cable crossovers does not even approximately reverse the fact that they are, overall, an inferior exercise. Compound exercises should nearly always be considered superior for building mass.

Ultimately, the issues of friction of machines and useless energy expenditure from balancing weights are minor and for the most part, inconsequential. To properly train some body parts (like hamstrings), machines *must* be used. For others (like chest), machines are optional. As long as the guidelines for generally favoring compound exercises and training with proper intensity are met, the decision to use one or the other comes down to personal preference. I have had excellent results from both. As evidenced by the particular training routines of various champion bodybuilders, either can be used to build a good deal of mass, and indeed, either can be used to become ultimately massive. Every single living champion bodybuilder uses a combination of the two.

Range of motion

It is important to use as full a range of motion as possible for most exercises. However, it can be useful to occasionally subject the muscles to a great deal of stress by using very heavy weights over a limited range of movement. This tactic is known as "partial reps." As with any advanced technique, the purpose should be to make the make the set being performed more difficult. But beyond the sheer added stress to the muscles, there are a couple of potential benefits to partial reps.

I will often begin pressing movements by performing several half-repetitions with the lower portion of the exercise; once I have reached a certain point (maybe five or eight reps), I will perform a few more reps using the full range of movement. The reason is this: As described in the section on pre-exhaustion, in many chest or shoulder pressing movements, the triceps will fatigue and reach failure first, before the larger target muscles. Much of this fatigue occurs in the top half of the range of motion, where the triceps seem to be doing more work. By performing half-reps first in the lower range, I am subjecting my chest or shoulders to a great deal of stress without causing inordinate and self-defeating fatigue to the triceps. When I reach the point where I begin the full-range reps, my chest or shoulder muscles have become more greatly fatigued than my triceps.

I also regularly perform a different type of partial reps—this time in the upper portion of the range of motion—for leg presses. My posture on most of my leg press sets makes this necessary. To avoid lower back problems, I keep my hips firmly planted against the back pad of the press, and I arch my back. I also place my feet together up high on the platform, as this increases the "feel" I get on my upper and outer thighs. When I lower the weight, my thighs are forced to stop when they reach my rib cage, hence the short range of motion. To compensate for the short range of motion, I use very heavy weights. However, the greatest benefit to this arrangement is that my knee joints endure relatively little stress. Knee problems are fairly common with weightlifting, so this is no small concern for lifters aspiring to avoid eventual disablement.

Exercises for the thighs that involve a full range of motion, squats in particular, are very effective and all-but-essential for growth. However, the combination of the full range of motion, hard work, very heavy weights, and high volume has spelled disaster for more than a few bodybuilders, as many have severe knee pain. In the worst cases, some have suffered a quadriceps tear, which is a particularly gruesome and disabling injury. The more common tears of the chest and biceps are horrible as well, but at least with those you can still walk. A quadriceps tear (which tends to come in pairs, since a tear on one leg during a pressing-type exercise will cause the other leg to immediately compensate by bearing all the weight, with the sudden extreme stress creating the second tear) will require the victim to be bed-ridden and wheelchair-bound for many months. As mentioned, using a full range of motion is necessary for optimum growth, but volume must be kept in check to insure longevity and avert disaster. And as is the most important point of this book, low-volume training is superior anyway.

Exercises

Quadriceps

Squats

This is the best mass-building exercise for the thighs and glutes, and indeed the best mass-building exercise ever devised. More than once squats have been referred to as the "king of exercises." Two points must be kept in mind with this exercise:

1. They must be performed with correct form.
2. They must be performed with immense intensity of effort.

It is very common to see squats being performed with bad form. Apart from the high risk of injury, bad form will also greatly limit the effectiveness of the exercise. The back must be kept tightly arched throughout the movement, with the head up. Apart from that, the subject needs to descend all the way to, or slightly above, the "parallel" position where, as the name implies, his thighs are roughly parallel to the floor. Also, it is important to "drive" the weight with the heels, not with the balls of the feet. Raising the heels off of the floor will cause a break in form and will add a great of stress to the knee joint.

More so than with any other exercise, the subject's performance with a set of squats is dictated by the amount of raw effort, of energy and determination, he is able to bring. With squats, greater effort can always result in more reps and therefore better results. This is unlike the case with many other exercises, where pitched intensity—albeit *always* having a good deal of worth—has a more limited value. For example, with the highest levels of motivation, a set of squats can be performed with a heavy weight for 20 reps—where you feel spent by the time the 12th rep is completed. When squatting with the right motivation, you can dig deep into your psyche and find the power to push on, and on, and on. And if you are able to do so, you *will* be rewarded.

A few other points:

1. Squats can be performed on a Smith Machine to good effect.
2. High-rep squatting is very effective. In my squatting heyday, the average number of reps I performed on working sets was higher than 20.
3. The width of stance should be determined by personal preference, essentially whatever is most comfortable. The notion that a particular stance should significantly influence the end result of pressing-type leg exercises has enjoyed a level of popularity that has far surpassed the value of the idea. Stance isn't that important.
4. Very hard leg training sessions, especially workouts that feature squatting, tend to have an overall anabolic effect on the body. Some research has shown that hard leg training will cause the body to release higher levels of testosterone and growth hormone, resulting in larger muscles everywhere. I personally noticed a sizable increase in overall mass once I began training my lower body in earnest. Every gym on the planet has a large number of members that do not train their legs, or that do so without a respectable level of effort. Over the years I have seen hundreds, maybe thousands of these. Not one has ever impressed me with his upper-body development. One might think that the extra energy that these people are conserving by avoiding leg training could be channeled into more productive upper-body workouts. It doesn't work that way. Hard leg training is necessary, and due to its extremely taxing nature, it can come about only through superior character and work ethic—with a superior overall physique as the reward. If you are not willing to endure brutal leg workouts, do not expect much success in bodybuilding.

Leg press

This is the second-best quadriceps exercise. Squatting involves the use of a greater number of muscle fibers, so leg presses will always play second fiddle. But leg presses are safer for the knees and especially the back.

Combined with the fact that they provide a decent level of effect, leg presses can be a passable choice as a primary leg exercise. More than a few top bodybuilders have used leg presses as the primary exercise for their quads, with no squatting. I myself made the decision to do so because of the safety factor (after almost a quarter-century of weightlifting, longevity is a very important concern), and also because I had built a good foundation as a result of years of *very* hard squatting.

Hack squats

Hack squats are considered to be the third-best quadriceps exercise. They have a tendency to be very hard on the knees, so unless the subject feels (or better yet, has evidence) that his particular structure benefits greatly from the movement, leg presses are a better choice: In general, they are less destructive to the knees and more effective.

Leg extensions

Leg extensions directly stress the front of the quads, in particular the lower area. The idea that performing leg extensions will cause greater or sharper definition is erroneous, as no exercise has this capability. The benefit of leg extensions is precisely the same as all single-joint exercises: They allow the subject to fully isolate the muscle being trained.

Thigh adductors

This exercise is one of the best-kept secrets in the world of leg training. Strong inner-thigh muscles add a good deal of stability when squatting. From a visual standpoint, legs that do not feature a full inner thigh will always appear somewhat scrawny. Adductors are an extremely effective exercise for building the inner thighs. Women seem to find far greater value in this exercise than men, since at least 90% of the people you will see performing this exercise are female.

Rotary-hip kicks

This exercise is another very well-kept secret; in fact, I very rarely see anyone other than myself performing these. A large number of gyms nowadays have a rotary-hip machine. This exercise is performed by placing the pad in front of the leg, slightly above the knee, and "kicking" the leg forward. To imagine how this works, stand in an upright position, and lift one knee as high as possible (it is okay to bend the knee). This exercise directly isolates the vastus intermedius and sartorius muscles. It is thought that leg extensions most effectively stress the front of the thigh, but with that exercise, much of the load is absorbed by the vastus medialis (or "teardrop") and lateralis muscles—and in a more general sense, the lower portion of the quad. Rotary hip-kicks hit the upper quad. A combination of extensions and rotary-hip kicks is an extremely effective way to fully train the front of the thigh.

Sissy squats

This is a somewhat antiquated exercise; legend has it that it will help to enhance the definition in one's thighs. As pointed out previously, such ideas reside in the realm of exercise mythology. The exercise is initiated from a standing position. The idea is that the subject should bring his upper body as close to the floor as possible *without* bending at the hips. In other words, one should be able to draw a straight line from his knees to his head, and this line should not bend or be broken throughout the exercise. This being the case, the knees will travel forward, and the thighs and upper body will tilt backwards, sort of like a limbo dance. Once the bottom position is reached, often when the shoulders are little more than a foot off the floor, the subject should ascend to the start position, again keeping the thighs and upper body in a stiff line. This movement is very difficult to perform without holding on to something to keep balance, such as one of the posts of a power rack; during the exercise, the hand will slide up and down it—for the purpose of balance, and also for self-assistance, if needed.

1. The good: Sissy squats are hard! It is a pretty good exercise if you ever find yourself wanting to work your legs without any access to weights or exercise equipment. This movement also fully isolates the quads.
2. The bad: This movement will not improve definition, and it is inferior to a combination of the leg extension and rotary-hip kick exercises.
3. The ugly: Sissy squats can be very hard on the knees.

Lunges

The main benefit of lunges is that they allow for a very large range of motion. The downside is that all of the muscles being worked with lunges can be more effectively trained using a combination of other exercises. Also, lunges have the potential to be hard on the knees. They are a good choice if the subject would like to get in a good upper-leg workout but not much weight is available.

A very popular iteration of the exercise is known as "walking lunges," in which the subject, with a weight on his shoulders, will take a giant step forward, descend into a full lunging position, and then stand straight up at the position of the forward foot. He then takes another step forward and lunges, this time with the other leg. He will therefore travel forward, hence the "walking lunge" description. Lunges are not terribly effective, and walking lunges are even less so. Due to the alternating execution of the movement, each leg gets to rest between each repetition—so there is no real constant time under tension. That, along with the relatively casual nature of the exercise itself, places a limitation on the level of intensity the subject can impose. As we have seen, the higher the intensity, the greater the growth.

Hamstrings

Leg curls

Leg curls are the primary exercise for the hamstrings. There are three main types: Lying, sitting, and standing. The decision of which one(s) to use is mainly a matter of personal preference. For example, I don't get a good "feel" from the standing variety, so I don't use them. However, I use both the lying and sitting variations, as I feel that there is enough difference between the two to warrant this choice. The lying type seems to stress the entire hamstring very well, while the sitting variety works the outer portion and the sartorius.

Stiff-legged deadlifts

Although this is an exercise very commonly incorporated into a hamstring workout, stiff-legged deadlifts are actually far more effective for the glutes and lower back. This type of deadlifting can indeed make the hamstrings very sore, and soreness is commonly and incorrectly equated with optimum growth-stimulation. Since stiff-legged deadlifts involve little or no bending at the knees, obviously the hamstrings will not be trained through a full range of motion—or *any* range of motion, for that matter. Rather, they are being tensed and stretched while under a sometimes considerable load. This will make them sore, but any growth of the hamstrings will be a result of other exercises.

To demonstrate the effectiveness of the exercise, consider the analogy of the following movement: Perform a barbell front raise, keeping the arms perfectly straight, *with your palms up.* Without bending the arms, raise the barbell until it is directly overhead. Then lower it through the same range of motion, and repeat. Now imagine that this is supposed to be a biceps exercise. The biceps might get very sore from this, but it is thoroughly working the shoulders, *not* the biceps. Likewise, stiff-legged deadlifts work the glutes and not the hamstrings. In fact, due to the bending of the knees, regular or especially sumo-style deadlifts are much better for stimulating growth in the hamstrings.

Also, stiff-legged deadlifts are dangerous, and some bodybuilders have suffered hamstring tears during this movement. As a glute movement it has value, but there are safer and more effective exercises for the glutes. Nevertheless, this movement is acceptable for females, for two reasons:

1. Women have a mechanical structure that is different from men, especially in the hip area, which allows for a safer and more effective execution of the exercise (although it should still not be considered a hamstring exercise).
2. Women appear to have a much lower risk of weightlifting-related injury. Studies have shown that women have a significantly higher risk for ligament tears in competitive sports[22], but the gym to seems to be safe ground. Faced with a lack of direct research to support this, however, I'll have to rely on anecdote: I have never known of any female weightlifter or bodybuilder that has suffered a complete muscle tear while lifting weights. That type of injury appears to be entirely the domain of men.

Men should avoid this exercise at all costs.

Glutes

Machine kickbacks

This is another exercise performed almost exclusively by women, and it is essentially another well-kept secret. It is a very effective way to train the glutes, which should be trained like all other muscles. Many bodybuilders figure that they will adequately train the glutes by performing squats and leg presses. These exercises do work well for stimulating growth in the glutes, but machine kickbacks isolate the muscle and are necessary for optimum effect.

They are performed one of two ways: Either on a rotary-hip machine, with the pad behind the knee, or on a specialized machine, with the foot pushing rearward on a platform. The former allows for more direct isolation; using the specialized glute machine is actually *less* specialized, since it is a compound-type movement. With these machines, the plate is pressed rearwards, involving the quads as well as the glutes. This is not necessarily bad, since the machine is constructed so that most of the stress will be on the glutes. But since we should imagine that the quads will have been optimally trained during their own session, there is no sense in subjecting them to additional, undue, and possibly detrimental stress. Also, the glute machine does place additional stress on the knees, which really can take only so much stress. Kickbacks on the rotary-hip machine do not stress the knees at all. Overall it seems that rotary-hip kickbacks are more effective, and they certainly conserve the knee joints.

Abductors

This is the final exercise which is almost exclusively the domain of women. It works the glutes in a somewhat different way from kickbacks, and tends to place greater stress on the upper and outer portion of the muscle. I have found it to be very effective, and anyone interested in fully training the glutes should consider incorporating this exercise.

Calves

Donkey and standing calf raises

There are three main types of calf raises: Standing, seated, and "donkey." All three types are effective. Donkey calf raises include three sub-types, the first of which being the original version, invented long before the advent of the donkey machine. This involves standing with the balls of the feet on a block, with the lower body perpendicular to the floor. The subject is bent forward at the waist, leaning on an immovable object, with his upper body roughly parallel to the floor. After assuming this position, he has someone sit on his back, as if that person were riding a donkey (hence the name). Without bending his knees, or maybe bending them only slightly, the subject lowers his heels as far as possible, then raises them up as high as they will go.

The second version involves the use of the machine intended to be used for this purpose, the so-called donkey calf machine. The most recent iteration sort of resembles a very short hack squat machine, with a pad only for the hip area. Rather than driving the resistance pad straight up, as is the case with the regular donkey machine, the subject drives it upwards and backwards at about a 45-degree angle, just like a hack squat.

The last version involves using a leg press machine. These are often referred to as "calf raises on a leg press machine," but for all intents and purposes, they are donkey calf raises, just performed in a slightly different position. What make this so is the fact that the resistance is placed on the hips, and not the shoulders, as is the case with standing calf raises. And, of course, they have the same effect as other versions of donkey raises. For that matter, they have just about the same effect as standing raises. For this reason, donkey raises are a better choice, because standing raises involve placing all of the weight on the spine.

Unless the subject somehow gets a significantly better "feel" from the standing version, donkeys are the way to go. It is never a good idea to needlessly subject the spine to heavy stress and pressure. For the young, enthusiastic, and carefree subject, this will seem a non-issue. However, anyone wanting to pursue bodybuilding for the "long haul" should make preservation of joints and connective tissue a top priority. The spine in particular should be treated with care. A single major back or joint injury, or less-catastrophic but collectively significant wear-and-tear, can impair or destroy that individual's efforts—and ultimately, his physique. Standing calf raises certainly aren't the worst thing you can do to your spine, but they will contribute wear-and-tear to a biological device that can only take so much.

Seated calf raises

This exercise isolates the soleus muscle. This exercise can be used if the subject is not getting adequate results for the soleus from donkey or standing calf raises alone. One problem with training the soleus, and indeed calf training in general, is that (perhaps more so than any other muscle) genetics play a huge role in determining the end result. Some people are born with massive calves, and some are barely able to add an inch of circumference. A few in the latter category are otherwise extremely muscular.

Back

Deadlifts

Deadlifts, like squats, can be brutally hard and remarkably effective. Many swear by deadlifts, but at the same time, there are a fair number of top bodybuilders that do not use them. They are highly recommended but ultimately not necessary. Although primarily considered to be a back exercise, deadlifts work a very large number of muscles, including all muscles of the upper leg, the glutes, and of course forearms (due to the tremendous gripping requirements—though most bodybuilders will use lifting straps whilst performing deadlifts). Some also feel that deadlifts have the full-body anabolic effect that comes with very hard leg training. On the negative side, deadlifts can be dangerous for the lower back, so proceed with caution.

Hyperextensions

These can be a fair substitute for deadlifts if the subject is not able to perform them. This exercise also directly isolates the lower back, which in itself has some value, but in no way should hyperextensions be considered a direct and equal replacement for deadlifts. However, they are safer, and all the muscles that are hit hard in a good deadlift workout will be trained directly in other sessions (quads being trained in a separate session being an example). Hyperextensions are also far safer than the other two exercises that directly isolate the lower back: Stiff-legged deadlifts and "good mornings."

The problems with stiff-legged deadlifts are discussed in the hamstrings section. As for good mornings, which are performed by bending forward at the hips while standing upright, all the while holding a barbell high on the back—it's not difficult to imagine that this exercise invites a high probability for injury. Also, in what should be the fully contracted position, the subject is standing upright; the weight is born on the on the spine, and the lower back muscles need exert little effort. With hyperextensions, the highest point in the movement is also the point of peak contraction for the lower back, a more effective compromise.

Rowing movements

These include dumbbell and barbell rows, as well as a variety of machine and cable rows. The primary purpose of these exercises is to add thickness to the back muscles. More than a few people believe that, of the bunch, barbell rows are the most effective. Meanwhile, many bodybuilders prefer machines for this purpose. And since there is no shortage of people with very good back development who do not incorporate barbell rows, one must conclude that they are not a necessity.

One problem with barbell rows is that there are only two possible hand positions: Overhand and underhand (fully-supinated). When using a normal (approximately shoulder-width) grip, the overhand position naturally causes the elbows to point outwards. This is opposite of what is ideal. The elbows should point inwards, toward the body, during rowing movements—and in the fully-contracted position, the subject should imagine trying to touch his elbows together behind his back. Of course, unless the subject is extremely flexible (and *not* very muscular), this is impossible. But the idea of attempting to touch elbows while squeezing the back muscles should give a good idea of what the fully-contracted position should feel like.

Some have sought to remedy this problem by using an underhand grip. This definitely solves the problem of achieving an ideal contracted position; the elbows point inwards, allowing the back muscles to contract to their fullest. However, the fully-supinated position places much more of a load directly on the biceps (it is for this reason that straight-bar curls are optimal for isolating that muscle). As has been mentioned, the biceps are fragile and susceptible to tearing. Dorian Yates found this out the hard way when he tore his biceps while performing underhand-grip barbell rows.

The brachialis muscles are considerably more durable, and to my knowledge, no bodybuilder or weightlifter has ever torn this muscle. As the degree of grip changes from the fully-supinated underhand to the overhand positions, the biceps become increasingly less involved (the brachialis more so), with very little involvement in the latter. Machines and cable attachments have a variety of such grip positions, so there need not be a choice between one of the two extremes. For example, seated cable rows are usually performed with a V-handle, which places the hands so that they are exactly halfway between the two extremes of rotation. This grip is both safe for the biceps and effective for allowing the elbows to squeeze inward as they travel backward. Machines have a variety of grip positions, depending on the particular model.

Machine rows have two further advantages:

1. It is easier to use certain high-intensity techniques with machines. Rest-pause and forced reps are accomplished more easily than with barbell rows.
2. Most machines are safer for the lower back. Barbell rows place the lower back in potential jeopardy, since it can be easy with this exercise to break form—and a break in form while bent-over at the waist and handling many hundreds of pounds can spell disaster for the subject. To be fair, T-bar rows (which is a machine exercise) can be nearly as dangerous.

For the most part, choices regarding which particular rowing exercises to use should be a matter of personal preference. Rows are compound movements, so they are essential for building a good deal of mass. As long as the chosen exercise is employed with sufficient intensity and the subject is mindful of the need for progression and adequate recovery, there are quite a few machines that can be used to good effect.

One-arm dumbbell rows are both safe and fairly effective, but some people find it difficult to get a good feel from this exercise. Also, nearly everyone employing this movement uses additional rowing exercises, so there can be a danger of redundancy of effect—which can be detrimental. One-arm dumbbell rowing is a decent exercise overall, but there are better choices. Also, there are one-arm rowing machines that are very effective, and essentially mimic the effect of the dumbbell movement.

Pulldown movements

Unlike rowing movements, which are meant to add thickness to the entire back, pulldown movements are used to increase lat width (since the downward-pulling motion heavily involves the lats but no so much the spinal erectors and other muscles of the back). Chins fall under this category; they are essential the free-weight version of pulldowns, and increasing the resistance of the movement typically involves hanging weight from the waist.

One common misconception is the idea that width of grip one uses in pulldowns or chins will ultimately determine the width of his lat development. Actually, it is a full-range of motion in the exercise, including a squeezed peak contraction at the bottom of the movement that will allow for such development. Very wide grips do not allow for a full range of motion, and essentially they will act to limit the development of one's lats, not enhance it. A medium, comfortable grip tends to be ideal for maximum lat stimulation.

Pulldowns can also be performed so that their effect more closely resembles that of a rowing motion. This is typically the case with close-grip pulldowns. This exercise has a slightly different effect than rowing movements, and it is generally safer. However, a popular method of performing close-grip pulldowns is by using an underhand grip on a straight bar, as it is relatively easy to get a good "feel" for the back by using such a grip (as mentioned above). I have never heard of anyone tearing a bicep while performing this particular exercise, but it should be kept in mind that any underhand or fully-supinated movement that involves bending and straightening the arms will add to accumulated wear-and-tear on the biceps and their tendons. Since biceps tear fairly easily, any unnecessary stress to that muscle should be avoided. Damage does accumulate, and muscles do eventually tear.

Pullovers

Pullovers isolate the lat muscles. This exercise can be valuable because there are few isolation movements for the back. For most people the back is the most difficult muscle to "feel" while training, and this gives pullovers extra value: They can be used in the first portion of pre-exhaustion set, or they can be employed as the first exercise of back workout—which can help to insure that the back muscles are "felt" and therefore trained properly. If the subject does not get a good feel for his back exercises, his arms and shoulders will end up bearing the brunt of the workout. And naturally, his back development will suffer.

Those without access to a pullover machine have two options: Straight-arm cable pushdowns and dumbbell pullovers. Cable pushdowns are the better choice of the two, for the following reasons:

1. Dumbbell pullovers have a shorter range of motion, because the arc of travel of the dumbbell cannot surpass the directly vertical position. This can be remedied somewhat by performing the exercise on a decline bench, although the bottom, stretched position of the exercise will be shortened.

2. At the very top portion of the dumbbell movement, tension on the lats is minimal, since the weight is essentially just being balanced at arms' length. With the cable movement, the lats will be subject to tension throughout the exercise.

3. Dumbbell pullovers naturally require a very narrow grip, which places a good deal of the stress of the exercise on the chest. For this reason, dumbbell pullovers are often thought of mainly as a chest exercise. This problem can be mainly fixed by performing the exercise with a short barbell or EZ-curl bar.

This is good example of a machine exercise being more effective than its free weight counterpart. The problem with both exercises is that they can considerably fatigue the triceps, despite the fact the fact that the arms are meant to be kept straight or almost so throughout the movement. Pullovers on a specialized pullover machine do not have this problem; since the resistance pad is driven by the upper arms.

With the dumbbell option, one other point bears mentioning: Many subscribe to the idea that dumbbell pullovers will increase the size of the rib cage. Some have gone so far as to recommend performing a superset of squats and dumbbell pullovers, the idea being that the labored, deep breathing resulting from the squats combined with the supposed rib cage-stretching property of pullovers will have the effect of increasing rib cage volume. As obvious as this may seem, it should be considered that the rib cage itself is nothing more than bone and connective tissue, and the shape and length of these items cannot be influenced by weightlifting exercises. Since the traditional "science" of weightlifting seems to have been formulated mainly by hunches and non-theoretical and uncontrolled experimentation, it can be easy to see how a nonsensical idea like this might enjoy some popularity.

Chest

Pressing movements

The employment of pressing movements is the key to building mass in the pectoral muscles. In spite of the popularity of fly-type exercises, they do little to increase mass. This being the case, it is normally a good idea to structure a chest workout around two types of presses: Inclines, as well as flat or decline presses.

Inclines place more direct stress on the upper (and harder to build) portion of the chest. A 30-degree angle is generally considered to be ideal. These can be performed with a barbell, dumbbells, or on a number of machines. The decision to use barbells or machines is discussed in the Free Weights vs. Machines section (p. 126). Regarding dumbbell presses, there are advantages and disadvantages as well. Dumbbell presses allow the most complete range of motion of all the choices (although you will often see people performing partial repetitions with dumbbells, which of course negates the one distinct advantage of the exercise); the subject can get a very good stretch at the bottom of the movement, and can get achieve a full contraction at the top by holding the dumbbells close together. A popular though useless technique is smacking the weights together at the very top of the movement. To set the record straight, this does not translate into greater growth—and it serves to weaken the dumbbells, which *will* break given enough abuse. (Spend enough time in gyms and you will realize that many techniques are both popular and useless.)

The primary disadvantage of dumbbell presses is that the number of high-intensity tactics that can be used is limited. For example, rest-pause can be very difficult with dumbbell presses, unless the subject has two training partners that are willing and able to hold the weights for him during the brief rests.

Perhaps the most popular exercise of all time is the flat bench press. It can be a very good mass-builder, but a number of people get better development from other exercises. One reason for this might be that flat benches tend to have a short range of motion. Dumbbells and certain machines are not so restricted. Also, bench presses can be very dangerous. More pecs are torn during the flat bench movement than seemingly all other chest exercises put together. In fact, anecdotes suggest that complete pec tears might be exclusively the domain of the flat bench press.

Apart from the obvious catastrophe of a pec tear, flat bench presses endanger the rotator cuff. Indeed, a large amount of stress is endured by the shoulder joints while performing flat presses. The reason for this is that the weight being lifted does not travel in a plane that includes the shoulder joints. This is not the case with inclines and declines, where the shoulder joint *is* in the plane of movement; in other words, in both of these exercises, the weight descends directly towards, and ascends directly away from the shoulder joint. This is not the case with flat benches, and the shoulder joint is strained significantly as a result. Some people are not bothered by this, and never have any problems benching. Anyone falling into this category, and who has also achieved a good deal of development from flat benches, is encouraged to use them. However, the flat bench press is by no means a necessary ingredient of a mass-building routine.

Decline presses, apart from being safer, are often more effective. As with flat benches, a relatively short range of motion is the main problem with the barbell version. This problem is not as easily remedied with dumbbells as in the case of inclines, since entering and exiting the decline position with heavy dumbbells can be difficult. Machine presses are effective, safe, and all high-intensity tactics can be used with them.

Dips also fall into the pressing movement category for chest, although they place a great deal of stress on the triceps and with a narrow grip are considered to be a triceps exercise. In general, dips can be a very good mass-building exercise, and they top the list of exercises that are both beneficial and can be performed when no weights are available (although, of course, dips bars or something similar will be needed). Like flat benches, dips can be very hard on the shoulder joint, so proceed with caution.

Flying movements

Being an isolation exercise, flyes have both the typical positive and negative qualities associated with such movements: On the plus side, they allow the subject to fully "feel" the muscle being trained; on the negative side, they are not good for building mass. Regarding the former, the ability to isolate and fatigue the muscle can be fully exploited through the pre-exhaustion technique. With the latter, it should be noted that flyes are not necessarily completely useless when used in a non-pre-exhaustion set. Machine flyes can allow for there to be full resistance at the peak, fully-contracted portion of the movement. Presses do not fully allow for this. Many bodybuilders will employ machine flyes or cable-crossovers in order to insure full development of the inner pecs.

However, a large number of bodybuilders will use crossovers or flyes as a means to "chisel" striations into the chest muscles. This idea is incorrect, as no exercise has the ability to increase definition by itself. Bodybuilders achieve these striations by reducing their body fat levels through dietary means. Often times, during a pre-contest phase, their weight-training workload will increase to include (or increase the number of) flyes. They mistakenly conclude that the flyes were the cause of (or a contributing factor to) the increased definition.

Flyes should not be considered an elemental part of a mass-building routine. The discussion of isolation exercises (p.125) made mention of the popularity of the cable-crossover movement. The fact that nearly all the people who religiously perform this exercise have sparsely-muscled physiques should be a clue as to its effectiveness. Beyond the anecdotes, however, the idea that compound movements almost always markedly trump isolation types as effective mass-builders can be recognized as the cause for the absence of real growth.

Shoulders

Pressing movements

The primary basic movement for the shoulders is the military press—a very effective movement. Behind-the-neck presses are also excellent, and allow for greater stimulation of the medial (middle) head of the deltoid. Some people find behind-the-neck presses to be uncomfortable, and in fact there is a greater chance of incurring a strain of one of the neck or upper-back muscles with this movement. Performing both exercises can have a redundant and potentially counterproductive effect. A choice between the two should be a matter of personal preference, as excellent deltoid development can result from the use of either.

Barbell presses do not have the same range-of-motion issues found with chest exercises, so from this standpoint machines do not present a clear advantage. But as always, machines allow for more possibilities with high-intensity tactics. Dumbbell presses have the same advantages and disadvantages found with dumbbell chest movements.

Side laterals

Shoulder workouts should also include an isolation movement for the medial head of the deltoids, namely a version of the side lateral exercise. As is the case with leg curls for hamstrings, this is an instance where an isolation movement is effective, and for many, indispensable. This is also another instance where machine movements are superior to free weights, for three reasons:

1. Machines offer constant resistance throughout the range of motion. With free-weight side laterals, the lower portion of the movement involves less resistance, since the weight does not ascend a great deal; in the higher portions of the movement, where the arms are roughly parallel to the floor, moving the weight one inch in the range of motion of the exercise requires lifting it approximately one inch higher. In the lower portion,

moving the weight one inch in the range of motion of the exercise might involve actually lifting it only a small fraction of an inch. In other words, much less force is required for this portion. With machines, the same amount of force must be applied to move the weight at any part of the motion.

2. Machines require the subject to sit down, which eliminates the tendency to initiate momentum of the weight with the knees, which is a very common tendency with this exercise. Of course, performing free-weight laterals whilst sitting eliminates this problem. Overall, machines make it easier to use strict form.

3. Machines for the most part make it easier to use high-intensity tactics.

Rear laterals

Like the middle section, rear deltoids also benefit a good deal from certain isolation exercises. These can be performed bent-over with dumbbells, on specific rear delt machines, or facing backwards on a pec-dec (machine flye) machine. The problems with the free-weight version are mainly the same as with side laterals. Nevertheless, in one effective variation, the subject lays face-down on an incline bench (at about 30 degrees) and performs the laterals with dumbbells—although this particular style often involves the use of much heavier dumbbells that can be used is a strict lateral fashion. The movement somewhat resembles a rowing exercise for the back, although the elbows are kept outward, away from the body—which is a departure from proper back-training form, which specifies that elbows should be travel inward during the exercise. The outward-pointing technique insures that the rear delts will absorb most of the stress of the exercise.

Front laterals

This exercise is meant to isolate the front delts. Unless the subject for some reason has a difficult time feeling his front delts during military or behind-the-neck presses, front laterals (or "front raises") are not particularly useful. As a matter of fact, considering all the work performed by the front delts throughout an entire full-body training cycle (*all* pressing exercises hit the front delts), front laterals are more likely to hurt than help, for the following four reasons:

1. The subject risks over-working the front delts.
2. Performing *any* unnecessary exercise impinges upon the subject's ability to recover.
3. The subject imposes unnecessary wear-and-tear on his shoulder joint.
4. The subject needlessly expends energy that could be used on better exercises.

In truth, if one were to set aside specific references to shoulder joints and muscles, these points apply to all redundant weightlifting exercises. One additional problem is caused by the fact that the more popular dumbbell version of the exercise is almost always performed in an alternating fashion. Due to this right-left alternating style, each delt is allowed to rest after each and every repetition—and this is exactly the same problem as with the walking lunges exercise. Front raises are sometimes performed with a barbell, which solves this issue, although the other problems remain.

Upright rows

As in the case of front laterals, unless the subject gets an especially good feel from this movement, it should be avoided. It will provide no special benefit beyond what can be achieved with presses and laterals. Regarding the former, it should be kept in mind that one can always push with greater force than he can pull; more weight can be moved through pressing exercises, and the subject need not worry about his grip tiring, as can happen with upright rows. But among those employing the movement, upright rows are never meant to replace presses, only compliment them. Essentially then, upright rows become a redundancy, the negative attributes of which being the same as with front laterals. Some people feel that upright rows hit the traps hard, but this effect should be seen as a redundancy of shoulder presses, most back exercises, and of course shrugs.

Shrugs

Shrugs isolate the traps. Some people like to go extremely heavy when performing this exercise, but end up bouncing the weight, using the legs to help with momentum, "hitching" the weight (partially resting it on parts of the body), and using a minimal range of motion. None of these things are good. It's a much better idea to use lighter weights (although "light" is a relative term here, since light shrugs might still involve fairly substantial poundages) that can be fully controlled through a full range of motion. Also, a straight up-and-down motion is ideal. The popular practice of rolling the shoulders forwards or backwards while reps are being performed will not create better results, and adds slightly to the possibility of injury.

Biceps

Barbell curls

This is overall a decent mass-building exercise. For optimum effect, a straight bar must be used; a cambered EZ-curl bar will reduce the work actually being performed by the biceps, with the brachialis muscles performing a greater portion of the work. Since with this exercise the weight is traveling in an arc, there is proportionately less stress on the biceps throughout the upper and lower parts of the movement.

Dumbbell curls

Dumbbell curls allow the subject to fully concentrate on achieving the best possible contractions for the biceps, one side at a time. As with a few other exercises, dumbbell curls are often performed in an alternating fashion, which is not optimal. Sometimes the exercise is performed by lifting the dumbbells together, in tandem. If the subject gets a better feel from tandem dumbbell curls than straight barbell curls, then this exercise is a good option. Otherwise, barbell curls are a better choice, since the straight grip on the bar forces the subject to fully supinate his hands. Dumbbell curls are best performed one side at a time, using the free hand to grip an immovable object for stabilization.

Preacher curls

The free-weight version of this exercise allows the subject to place extra stress on different parts of the biceps, depending upon the configuration of the bench being used. Preacher benches, when viewed from the side, typically form a right triangle. In the standard version of the exercise, the upright section of the bench is in contact with the torso. The upper arms rest on the downward-sloped part of the bench. This exercise places a great deal of stress on the lower biceps, since the lower portion of the arc of travel of the barbell (or dumbbell) is closest to a vertical line. To contrast, with normal barbell curls, the lower portion involves more forward than vertical travel of the weight—hence less stress on the muscle in the lower segment.

However, with the standard version of preacher curls, there is little or no tension on the biceps in the top portion, since the forearms are virtually perpendicular to the floor, and the weight is mainly just being balanced there until the eccentric portion of the movement begins. The problem is the opposite with other version of preacher curls, where the subject leans against the sloped portion of the bench, and the arms hang down vertically. As one might guess, this version places more stress on the upper portion of the biceps, with far less stress on the lower. Actually, this exercise can be referred to as *preacher concentration curls.*

Many companies have sought to alleviate the problem of uneven resistance entirely by designing machines that allow for full and complete tension throughout the movement. Some of these machines can be very good, and the only problem is finding or having access to one that adequately suits the subject's unique mechanical structure. These machines typically should have a plate-loaded cable and cam system, since single-joint plate-loaded machines often do not fully address the issue of uneven resistance.

Dumbbell concentration curls

This exercise involves assuming a posture such that the upper body inclines forward, allowing the upper arm to hang downwards. This is most often achieved by sitting down, or by leaning against an immovable object with the arm not being trained. The sitting version typically involves resting the back of the arm being trained against the inner thigh on the same side of the body. In this posture, the exercise closely mimics the dumbbell version of the preacher concentration curl described above. The version where the arm is not supported by the subject's leg or a bench has a nearly identical effect, the main difference being that it is easier to use the cheating tactic. Concentration curls allow the subject to most effectively isolate the biceps, with a relatively large amount of tension available at the top of the range of motion.

Cable curls

Cable curls can be performed instead of free weights, with maybe a little more tension available for certain parts of the range of motion of the exercise. For example, preacher curls with a cable will place more stress on the biceps in the top of the range of motion, because the path of maximum resistance is not a vertical line, as is always the case with free weights. The path of resistance is a line from the handle at the end of the cable to the pulley of the weight stack. Often times this line is in the neighborhood of 45 degrees, depending of course upon the height of the preacher bench and the distance of the bench from the pulley. A 45-degree angle of resistance will place a great deal more stress at the top of the range of motion than will a free weight, but much less stress at the bottom. To contrast, machine preacher curls place fairly even resistance throughout the range of motion. Machine preacher curls are superior.

Certain isolation exercises occasionally enjoy "vogue" status. Cable crossovers, for example, have a degree of popularity that vastly overrates the effectiveness of the exercise. Rope-handle triceps pushdowns were once a very common site in a few of the gyms to which I previously belonged. (And it is worthy of mention that brutally hard exercises like squats and deadlifts, despite their unquestionable effectiveness, have always been very unpopular!) One exercise now in vogue is a version of cable curls that some like to call "crucifix curls." These are performed at a cable-crossover station (by now a very familiar locale for the people who tend to be attracted to this exercise); instead of performing crossovers, the subject, with palms up, performs curls so that his end posture resembles a "front double biceps" pose. One might think the people doing this exercise are more interested at looking at themselves in the mirror than trying to objectively assess the effectiveness of the exercise. This is another one that offers uneven resistance, and the mechanical particulars of the movement do not give it any type of advantage over conventional biceps exercises. However, if someone is currently using this exercise and purports to get a good feel from it, it wouldn't be unreasonable to continue its use. Otherwise, there is no reason to recommend it.

Triceps

Close-grip bench press

This is perhaps the best mass-builder for the triceps. Unlike regular flat bench presses, this exercise does not place the shoulder joint in peril. The grip need not be excessively close, and such grips strain the wrists anyway. The distance should be determined by comfort, and there should be a gap between the hands of six to twelve inches. Keeping the elbows close to the body ensures that the triceps will receive the maximum level of stimulation possible. Allowing the elbows to travel outward involves the chest more. This exercise is a good candidate for the second portion of a pre-exhaustion set.

Dips

This is another good mass-building exercise. Dips, when performed for the specific purpose of stimulating the triceps, bear a close resemblance to the chest exercise, except that typically (when possible) they are performed on bars that are closer together. This close spacing does not specifically enhance the stress applied to the triceps, but it does help to reduce involvement of the chest muscles. It is possible to become very strong with this exercise, such that weight must be attached to the waist in order to keep the rep range fairly low. A better alternative would be to pre-exhaust the triceps with an isolation exercise such as cable pushdowns first, for the following two reasons:

1. This will allow the subject to enjoy the benefits of the pre-exhaustion tactic (page 100).
2. This will cause less stress to the shoulder joint. The mere fact that pre-exhaustion will allow the subject to work just as hard without loading the extra weight (and therefore strain) on the joint will help to preserve the shoulder. As mentioned previously, an injury to the shoulder joint can be disastrous.

Dips can also be performed on specialized dip machines with plate-loaded resistance (with a belt that locks the subject in place). This machine is as effective as weighted dips, and much more convenient, since the subject doesn't need to affix a belt with weights dangling from it. It is equally hard on the shoulder joints, however, so caution should be observed.

A version of dips can also be performed with two parallel benches; the feet are propped on one, with the palms of both hands on the other, which is behind the back. These are commonly referred to as "bench dips." These can also be rather hard on the shoulders, even more so than regular dips. On top of that, they offer even less resistance than regular dips, since a fair amount of the subject's weight is resting on the foot bench. Nevertheless, they hit the triceps more directly than regular dips. It is common to add resistance by balancing weights on the lap during the exercise. As with regular dips, a better and safer idea is to employ the pre-exhaustion technique, with bench dips following an exercise like cable pushdowns.

Lying extensions

Lying extensions are a good exercise for the triceps, and are best performed with an EZ-curl bar. Unlike the case with biceps, where a straight bar is most effective, triceps are best trained with a cambered bar. The reason is mainly that a straight bar places greater stress on the wrist joints. This exercise is best executed by allowing the head to hang *slightly* off the end of a flat bench. This will allow the forehead to be a little lower than if the head were resting on the bench. In turn, this will allow for a slightly better range of motion for the exercise, since the bar is typically lowered to the forehead (hence the nickname for the exercise of "skull crushers"). It is also a good idea to lift this bar in a straight, vertical line from this point—not to a point where the arms are perpendicular to the floor—as this will insure that there will be constant tension on the triceps. When the arms are holding a weight in the vertical position, there is less tension on the triceps.

Behind-the-head extensions

These can be performed with a single dumbbell held by both hands, with a dumbbell held in one hand, or on a cable-pulley machine specifically designed for this exercise. This is a good isolation exercise that allows for a full range of motion.

Cable pushdowns

Cable pushdowns are the most popular isolation exercise for the triceps, and are probably the most popular triceps movement, period. They are also overrated, and many beginners can be seen performing endless sets of cable pushdowns, of every conceivable variety: Straight bar, cambered bar, rope handle, reverse grip, single-arm, the list goes on. This is unquestionably an effective and worthwhile exercise, but for triceps mass, one is better off performing close-grip benches and dips. Pushdowns are an acceptable elective exercise, or a good choice for the first part of a pre-exhaustion set. The determination of type of grip used (straight, cambered, V-handle, rope handle) should mainly be a matter of personal preference, as the idea that particular grips stress different parts of the triceps to a significant degree is overrated.

Dumbbell Kickbacks

This exercise affects the triceps in a manner similar to single-arm cable pushdowns, except that, due to the bent-over posture, the resistance is greatest at the very top (arms extended portion) of the range of motion. With pushdowns, resistance is greatest near the bottom (arms bent) part. This is another decent isolation exercise.

Forearms

Wrist curls

These are performed a few different ways, the most common being to rest both forearms, palms-up, on a flat bench. The hands ought to hang off the end, grasping a barbell. In this position, the hands are curled upwards as high as possible, towards the body, then lowered as far as they will go. As one might imagine, then range of motion of this exercise is very short. Another version calls for the same posture, except that this time the palms are facing downwards. Obviously this works the other side of the forearms. A third type involves a standing posture with a barbell held behind the body, and arms more or less held straight down. The subject, using an overhand grip, curls the hands upward. This works in inside forearm muscles is a somewhat similar way to the first example.

The good news is that it is possible and even common to achieve excellent forearm development without ever performing specific forearm exercises. Forearms are forced to work very hard during biceps and back workouts, even when lifting straps are involved. Of course, one way to insure that the forearms are trained very hard is to perform one or more back exercises *without* lifting straps.

However, for some people, this is not enough. Indeed, although the forearms must work very hard during certain exercises, only specific forearm exercises will subject them to optimum stress through a full range of motion. Beyond that, only during specific forearm exercises should the forearm muscles reach failure. If the forearms are reaching failure during back exercises, obviously this will impinge upon the effectiveness of the back workout, and straps should be employed to alleviate this—and forearm exercises should be included to bring their strength up to par. The short way of stating all of this is that one should only train forearms if he needs to; otherwise, they'll get plenty of stimulation through other exercises.

Hammer curls

Hammer curls are identical to regular dumbbell curls, except that the palms should remain perpendicular to the floor (as if one were swinging a hammer). This exercise is meant to train the upper forearm and brachialis muscles. Although this exercise is not a bad idea per se, these same muscles are subject to very intense contractions during a typical back workout. Inasmuch, this is literally an exercise in redundancy.

Reverse curls are very similar to hammer curls, the exception being that they are performed with a barbell and a reverse (overhand) grip. They mainly work the forearm and brachialis muscles in the same way as hammer curls. They have the same fundamental problem of redundancy. Neither is advisable unless the subject is suffering from exceptionally weak forearm development and is in need of some kind of boost in that area.

Abdominals

Hanging leg raises

Leg raises, performed hanging from a bar, are effective for training the entire abdominal area. They are also a good exercise because they are difficult. Contrary to what many people think, defined abdominals do not come about as a result of hammering out thousands of crunches. With hanging leg raises, a set just can't go on for very long, *because they're hard.* And performing a hard set that can't go forever is consistent with the idea that abdominals should be trained just like other muscles.

It just so happens that the abdominal area, at least for men, is where most fat is stored. Ages ago the myth was hatched that hours of abdominal work, performed daily, would be the key to removing that layer of fat. It is not. I know people that perform hundreds or even thousands of crunches daily—and somehow they still have this layer of fat. Granted, crunches *are* exercise, and any exercise will burn calories. And if you are able to burn more calories than you take in, you will lose fat. So in this sense, crunches can help get rid of the fat. But there is a far better way to go about it.

Endless crunches can easily lead to burnout. And thank goodness that exercise like this is not only not required—it is also not advisable. Would anyone really want to do a couple hours of crunches every day to get a defined waistline? The best way to go about it is to train abs with high intensity, about as frequently as any other body part. The much sought-after definition will come about as a result of having low bodyfat. To decrease bodyfat, the subject needs to burn more calories than he takes in. There are a few different strategies and tactics for reducing bodyfat in the most efficient manner, but those are beyond the scope of this chapter and really this book. The point here is that long, drawn-out abdominal workouts by themselves are a bad idea.

The question then becomes whether abs should be trained exactly as other body part. In training other body parts, the idea is to achieve the greatest degree of muscular growth possible. This is not the aim of abdominal workouts, and indeed, the abs are one muscle group that is not capable of dramatic growth. (The very large waistlines of some of today's top bodybuilders are a result of the growth of their internal organs from chemical enhancement, not from heavy ab training). That being the case, it is less important when training abs to adhere to a certain rep range or avoid any volume of training beyond what is required for growth stimulation. This is not to say that very high-volume ab workouts are a good idea, since superfluous work will unnecessarily impinge upon the body's general recovery abilities, affecting the subject's overall growth. A complete and effective ab workout can take less than five sets total, sometimes as few as two.

But the abs should be trained to failure, and a full range of motion should be used. This is why hanging leg raises are such a good choice. Unlike crunches, hanging leg raises cannot go on forever, so it won't take an eternity to reach failure. And when performed properly, the range of motion with this exercise is excellent. Because the exercise is performed hanging from a bar, there is a tendency to swing back and forth during the set. To make this exercise effective, there can be no swinging. A small degree of coordination is required in order to pull this off. Anyone that absolute cannot muster the coordination to not swing back and forth can substitute the version of the exercise performed on an upright bench designed specifically for this purpose. This variation is a little less effective, but overall it is still a very decent exercise.

Leg raises tend to add proportionately greater stress to the lower abdominal area, so it is often a good idea to compliment this exercise with an upper-ab movement such as crunches.

Crunches

As mentioned, sets of traditional crunches can go on for very long periods of time. This is because there is very little resistance in the exercise. And as described above in the principles of high-intensity theory, a set that is long in duration cannot be intense. Crunches do involve contractions of the entire abdominal wall, so they can be made a good exercise by adding resistance. Fortunately there are a variety of machines that accomplish this. Like leg raises, crunches work the entire abdominal wall. However, the latter tend to concentrate stress on the upper region of the abs, making them a good compliment to the former.

A version of crunches can also be performed with a rope handle on a pulldown cable. These might hit the abs in a slightly different way than machine crunches; also this is a very decent alternative if no crunch machine is available. Likewise, a type of crunches can be performed on an incline bench. A weight can be held in front of the chest for added resistance. This is also a decent exercise.

Twists

Twisting movements tend to work the sides of the waist: The obliques and intercostals, and to some degree the serratus, lats, and other muscles of the torso. Broomstick twisting is an exercise that has stood the test of time, and like many exercises and concepts that have been handed down through the ages, it resides in the realm of the nonsensical. After all, how long will it take to reach failure with a set of stick twists? Hours? Days? Any muscle worth training is worth training to failure. This is almost an impossibility with stick twists. As is the case with crunches, stick twists *are* exercise, and *will* burn calories. But a better idea would be to train the muscles that twists attempt to target with legitimate sets, taken to failure, and supplement the overall routine with some type of cardio exercise if extra calorie-burning or metabolism-boosting is desired. Performing the twisting exercise on a machine specifically designed for that purpose is an entirely different matter, since it is possible to use a high amount of resistance. With this exercise, sets can be taken to failure.

The main problem with exercises that target the sides of the waist is that they threaten to build up those muscles a good deal, which can detract from an aesthetic "V"-shaped upper-body taper. A hugely-muscled upper body looks all the more impressive when the waist is small. Mention was made of the fact that the abdominal muscles can be made larger by only a small degree. This is less so with the oblique muscles, which can grow enough to degrade the V-taper.

The oblique muscles should be trained just like all other muscles. However, a good deal of effort is often directed at this area by many lifters, as a disproportionate amount of fat is stored on the sides of the waist. These unsightly deposits are euphemistically referred to as "love handles." The idea is that the large amount of work will accelerate the removal of fat from the area. This concept is known as "spot reduction," and has been proven to be a myth. As has been mentioned a few times already, no exercise will, by itself, improve definition. On top of that, a standard abdominal workout, combined with complete training for the back and lower body, will provide sufficient training for this area. Ridding one's self of love handles is a function of diet.

Nutrition

A complete discussion of a proper bodybuilding diet is a subject for a complete other book. This purpose of this book is to discuss training for the specific purpose of building mass. Nevertheless, there are some basic concepts that should be considered:

1. Eat enough protein. A generally accepted rule-of-thumb is that bodybuilders should eat one gram of protein daily for each pound of bodyweight. Some have disputed this claim, saying that such an intake is excessive (while others advocate eating a far greater amount). Whatever the case, many have built a high degree of muscle mass by following this rule.
2. Eat several meals at even intervals throughout the day. The human body can only metabolize so much protein at a time. If the subject weighs 200 pounds, using the above guideline he will be consuming 200 grams of protein per day. If he eats all 200 grams in a single meal, most of it will go to waste; it will be excreted, stored as fat, or burned as energy. On the other hand, if he eats six meals per day, averaging 30-35 grams of protein per meal, he gives his body much more opportunity to convert that protein into muscle. Also, the most direct way to stimulate the metabolism is by eating. Eating every few hours keeps the metabolism moving; eating a small number of large meals slows down the metabolism, which will incline the body to store fat.
3. Allow for sensible ratios of macronutrients. It is reasonable to assume that a hard-training, 200-pound bodybuilder with a relatively low percentage of body fat can make good gains by consuming about 3200 calories per day. (Of course, there is a very wide range concerning what is ideal, depending upon the metabolic particulars of the individual; some will need more, some less). Since there are four calories per gram of protein, an individual eating 200 grams of protein per day will be eating 800 calories' worth of that macronutrient—or 25% of his daily calories. That leaves the other 75% to be distributed between carbohydrates and fats. It is sensible and effective to allow 60% of the entire compliment to be composed of carbs (480 grams; at four calories per gram, that's 1920 calories), the remaining 15%

being fats (53 grams; at nine calories per gram, that's 480 calories). It can also be okay to reduce carbs slightly, maybe down to 50%, while bumping up protein and fats (to something like 30 and 20 percent, respectively).

4. Carbohydrates are your friend. The carb-bashing of the last decade somehow found a solid footing in the bodybuilding community, despite the fact that carbohydrates are required to achieve full, hard-looking muscles. Low carbohydrate intake will cause the muscles to be flat and flaccid, and will make them weak. At the same time, however, all carbohydrates are not created equal. Refined sugar should be avoided as much as possible, since it will quickly be used as energy or stored as fat. The intake of refined sugar will also cause uneven blood sugar levels, resulting in periods of very high and very low energy levels. It is best to favor the intake of carbohydrates that do not cause rapid increases in blood sugar levels. Complex carbohydrates tend to fall into this category, as do most vegetables and fruits. Refined foods, especially including those high in sugar, tend to raise blood sugar levels quickly—with a corresponding "crash" afterwards—and should be avoided.

5. Be aware of your diet. I continue to be astonished by the number of aspiring bodybuilders that are unaware of the amounts of calories or macronutrients they are taking in. Worse still is the group of low-level bodybuilders that, even when preparing for competition, do not even know how many calories they are consuming on a daily basis. These people are universally dissatisfied with their results, and little wonder.

6. Be consistent. Proper nutrition is critical, but to get results, one must eat well; the less deviation, the better.

7. Drink lots of water. Muscle is 70% water. Plus, it's very healthy to do so.

8. Avoid "cheat days." Cheat days, which allow for the consumption of large amounts of junk food (usually on a weekly basis), are not a good idea. They will make you fat. Some feel that they help psychologically. They do not. They hurt psychologically. The idea that it is okay to eat for psychological purposes opens up a huge can of worms. One should endeavor to completely disassociate emotion from eating. Food should be viewed as a tool by which one can optimize his efforts and enjoy the best possible results. Falling in love with food or eating can only lead to bad

things, food obsession not be the least of these. This does not mean that one should not enjoy his food. Food can be very enjoyable. This is why there are so many fat people in all but the poorest of countries. But there are other things in life that enjoyable as well. Focus on these instead. Being in shape is one such pleasure. To paraphrase a recent 15-minute celebrity, "nothing tastes as good as being in shape feels." Consciously planning a cheat day is tantamount to admitting that your emotions control you, rather than the other way around.

The importance of nutrition should not be underestimated. There are many "three-legged stools" in life, and the specific elements of a mass-building regiment comprise such an arrangement. Whereas the whole of an individual can be divided into intellectual, emotional, and physical components, a similar arrangement exists in the relationship of training, nutrition, and rest. Some like to attach a percentage of importance to each of these factors. More than once I have heard it proclaimed that "bodybuilding is 80% nutrition." Obviously this leaves only 20% for training and rest. We'll humor this assertion by assuming that training will count for 10% and rest for the other 10%. This being the case, one could have perfect nutrition and optimum rest and—ignoring training altogether—he could still have a physique that would be 90% as good as its potential. Obviously this is nonsense. Nutrition is critical nevertheless. Nutrition, training, and rest are equally important. Ignore nutrition and poor results await.

IV

Intangibles

"What is steel compared to the hand that wields it?"
-Thulsa Doom

On War

"One might say that the physical seem little more than the wooden hilt, while the moral factors are the precious metal, the real weapon, the finely-honed blade."

When the Prussian military theorist Karl von Clausewitz set forth this declaration in his masterpiece *On War* in the early 19th century, he did not have bodybuilding in mind. But this idea, like much of what he wrote concerning moral factors in armed conflict, has found a direct application in the world of athletic performance and certainly weight training. After all, in some respects bodybuilding *is* warfare. Of course, in the realm of physique competition, one can be thought of as being at war with his competitors; this is true of any type of competition or sport, so the idea of embracing a warrior's mentality should not be foreign. But unlike nearly all sports which pit the performance of one athlete or team against another within the confines and criteria of the actual competition, bodybuilding is, in its entirety, a war against one's self. This being the case, that those determined to enjoy success in bodybuilding *are* at war, then it is valuable to investigate the comparison more closely.

The basic ingredients for success in both are the same. The idea that intellectual, physical, and intangible or "moral" factors all have a role to play in a successful mass-building campaign is implied by the very format of this book. This sentiment is also conveyed by the official United States Marine Corps' manual on combat and warfare *Warfighting*, which states the following (from chapter one, *The Nature of War*):

"Mental forces provide the ability...to make effective estimates, calculations, and decisions; to devise tactics and strategies; and to develop plans...War is characterized by the interaction of both moral and physical forces. The physical characteristics of war are generally easily seen, understood, and measured...The moral characteristics are less tangible...Moral forces are difficult to grasp and impossible to quantify...Because moral forces are difficult to come to grips with, it is tempting to exclude them from our study of war. However, any doctrine or theory of war that neglects these factors ignores the greater part of the nature of war."[23]

The analogy plainly conveys the idea that a well-planned physical effort enlisting moral factors of the highest order will yield the best results. As pertains to the individual soldier, the moral qualities specifically encompass discipline, energy, determination, and courage. The moral factors in weight training are identical. The manual later states the following:

"The object in war is to impose our will on our enemy."[24]

Here is where the distinction begins. In the gym, we are not directing attacks, forming pincer movements, or killing people. We are lifting weights. The context of the war of bodybuilding is of course different from actual war; it is a struggle to maintain ongoing motivation, and when need be, to markedly raise the level of that motivation. This may sound easy, certainly easier than engaging in a real killing contest. But the illusion of relative ease might help foster the high rate of failure. Also, real war brings with it an imperative of action: Kill or be killed—or if not killed, at least dominated and humiliated. The repercussions of failing at weight training are decidedly less severe. The decision to prevail is based on no such dire imperative, but rather on a commitment to the task, and to one's self. To prevail, both must be unassailable.

The act of markedly raising the level of motivation when required is necessary to insure the training sessions themselves are optimal, and bears analogy to the moral forces existing within battles themselves. (Having never participated in a real battle, I am forced to rely on the observations of the experts.) The other element, that of ongoing motivation, is obviously necessary for remaining dedicated to the undertaking. The entities that are the focus of the struggle for ongoing motivation include some of the basic driving forces of human behavior, namely human instincts.

Whereas much has been made of the idea of so-called "instinctive" training in relation to lifting weights, the war of bodybuilding is actually a war *against* instinct. Instinct tells us to avoid exertion unless it is absolutely necessary for survival. Weight training is not necessary for survival. The primary function of instinct is to help perpetuate the species through, among other things, self-preservation. Maintaining a sedentary posture at every opportunity is one way to insure self-preservation.

To alien observers, humans might appear to be primarily sedentary creatures. Most humans will exert enough physical effort required to survive—in first-world modern society this can be little or none—but beyond that, their lives are spent seeking pleasure. Some pleasures are readily available and easily obtained. Sitting on a couch in front of a television with a bag of potato chips is one such pleasure. It's not hard to imagine that very little effort is required to obtain this. The gratification is immediate. There is a downside to this pleasure, since activities like this will make you fat.

There are countless other human pleasures, one being the satisfaction of becoming fit. But unlike sitting on a couch, stuffing your face, the pleasure experienced from being fit is not easily obtained. In fact, it can be very difficult to achieve this. The gratification is delayed. The effort required to achieve fitness has often been described as a "battle." More accurately, it is an ongoing series of battles—hence part of the comparison to war.

By sitting on the couch and eating, the subject is staying out of harm's way, barricaded from the outside world and whatever dangers might lurk there. He is also resting and adding precious layers of fat that will come in handy when food is scarce. Of course, being first-world modern humans, almost none of us will ever experience a scarcity of food, so this becomes an exercise in sloth and gluttony, more modern concepts that arose from a more modern existence.

What is required then is a triumph of ego over the impulse to shelter oneself within the lowly basics of human existence. This concept is somewhat abstract and quite beyond the conscious planning of most committing to an exercise regiment. It is possible that this is part of the reason so many fail. But since humans are beings of dual nature, they have a side that is *not* content to merely exist; they have a force of will to seize upon, if it can be located and awakened. Humans may be slothful and gluttonous, yet they can also be fountains of volition, action, and desire. Ayn Rand, in *Atlas Shrugged,* characterized man as a "heroic being... with productive achievement as his noblest activity."[25] Friedrich Nietzsche, in *Beyond Good and Evil,* mainly concurred:

> "Physiologists should think before putting down the instinct of self-preservation as the cardinal instinct of an organic being. A living thing seeks above all to discharge its strength—life itself is will to power; self-preservation is only one of the indirect and most frequent results."[26]

I hold the pessimistic view that such sentiment applies to the few rather than the many, since many people never seem to achieve much more than reproducing themselves. But the duality remains. However latent, within each individual lies the power to be strong (in a figurative and literal sense), productive, even heroic. To realize this power, an internal war must be fought and won. Anyone faced with a general lack of motivation should seek help from experts in the area. Volition, action, and desire lurk beneath the surface in every human, but they must be invoked. Until such time as that can be accomplished, this book is likely not for them. It should also be realized that by no means is empowerment of the individual attainable only through weight training. The struggle between volition and instinct applies to all types of productive achievement.

For some people fighting the war is easy, as they have no shortage of motivation. These are the ones to whom Rand and Nietzsche must have been referring. And here is where things get slightly tricky: Training for the specific purpose of building mass is one rare instance of an undertaking that will be subverted by excessive effort—hence the lengths

I have gone to prescribe a strategy that will avoid this. A great reward of realizing and carrying out an efficient training regiment is that it leaves time for other worthwhile, even noble pursuits.

For people like this, the ones in possession of general determination and knowledge of the need to restrict their efforts, it only becomes a question of gathering motivation and focusing it, allowing it to all be released at one critical point, much like an explosion. In one sense, the idea of "imposing our will" means having the ability to create the highest levels of physical intensity possible, on demand. This is critical. High-intensity training does not require a great deal of time or a vast expenditure of energy. But for optimal results and by definition, it does require the ability to train—in brief and infrequent sessions—as hard as humanly possible.

Courage

Courage in the weight room is obviously quite different from courage on the battlefield. They are distant cousins, the kill-or-be-killed imperative of the latter being far and away the distinguishing factor. Besides the grunting and clanking of weights, gyms are peaceful places. Courage existing within a gym is far more subtle than putting one's life on the line; rather, it is the action of enthusiastically confronting physical pain and hardship. Advanced lifters who are capable of moving very heavy weights are well-acquainted with such courage. Many heavy basic exercises are quite uncomfortable and painful, and anyone executing such a set knew that this would be the case before the first repetition. Yet people lift like this every day. They don't do it when they're scared. When the time comes, they summon their courage, and they begin. If they cannot summon this courage, they fail. This is a simple concept.

Discipline

Discipline is the primary factor responsible for maintaining the ongoing motivation necessary for keeping the greater effort moving forward, though it is fueled by determination. Its role in this regard requires little explanation. But by the moment the weightlifting set commences, that form of discipline has played its part. A second type of discipline then becomes critical; that concerning the ability to induce a state of mental—and therefore physical—readiness. This is the discipline of thought.

The state of optimum mental and physical readiness is often referred to as "the zone," a somewhat catch-all term used to describe a temporary condition of supreme concentration and unimpinged immersion in the task at hand.[27] The zone state of mind seems to have a measurable physiological correlation. The activity level of human thoughts can be determined by measuring the oscillations of electromagnetic waves produced by human brains, otherwise known as "brain waves." Supreme concentration has been shown to occur when these waves are less busy, residing in the 8-12 Hertz range. These have been called "Alpha" waves, and persons with a high incidence of Alpha wave output include those practicing Buddhist Zen exercises and Yoga. Snipers have also been measured to have a higher degree of accuracy in their shooting when producing Alpha waves. For practical purposes, it can be assumed that we are producing Alpha waves when in a state of deep, uninterrupted concentration, without intrusive thoughts.[28] On the other side of this equation are Beta waves, which denote "the states associated with normal waking consciousness. Low amplitude beta with multiple and varying frequencies is often associated with active, busy or anxious thinking and active concentration."[29] Beta waves are present when the range of electromagnetic output exceeds 12 Hertz.

Obviously an ideal working set will take place when in a state of unimpinged mental immersion. Though it is not practical to attempt to accurately measure brainwaves during a training session, it is helpful to realize that there is a physiological correlation. It should be easy to tell when the activity is in the Beta range, simply because concentration is poor or fair and intervening or intrusive thoughts are being entertained. The Alpha phase will occur much less frequently, and typically it is something realized after the fact. Reflecting on a period of concentration and corresponding Alpha activity might cause one to deduce that the state had been attained. An optimum working set will consist of the mental discipline of concentration and a high level of energy.

Energy

Intense physical output requires a high level of energy, at least for the brief instance of the working set: The higher the better. Supreme concentration will create the physical state which will allow this. Concentration can in fact help boost the secretion of the hormone adrenaline. This is desirable, since adrenaline has two benefits: It has energizing and pain-killing effects—both handy attributes, especially the former. Adrenaline will temporarily elevate strength levels. It raises the supply of oxygen and glucose in the blood stream, directly boosting energy levels and therefore indirectly increasing strength. The mythical image of adrenalin-invoked strength is that of the woman lifting the Cadillac off of her trapped child.

The intended purpose of adrenaline is worthy of consideration. The human brain developed from rather less complex versions. The reasoning capacity of these early iterations matched their complexity. When faced with certain circumstances, there were two choices available: Fight or flight. Adrenaline is the flight-or-flight hormone, secreted when such situations arise. The sole purpose of any species is merely to perpetuate itself, and this can only be accomplished if its individual members place a premium on self-preservation. Mechanisms like fight-or-flight, combined with energy-boosting hormonal secretion, are in place to insure this. The self-preservation mechanism is hard-wired.

With the development of the human brain, there are now a far greater range of options, with an equally large continuum of nuance. Nevertheless, the fight-or-flight mechanism remains. Though it may be more of an impediment than benefit to majority of first-world modern humans, its effect can be exploited. It is exploited on the battlefield and in sporting arenas. It can also be exploited in the weight room.

The fight-or-flight mechanism is triggered by association. In lower animals, the association of danger can be through very simplistic interpretation. A snake will assume a defensive posture once it detects a large enough object within a certain proximity. It associates this object, whatever it is, with danger—and prepares to fight. Humans have vastly superior reasoning abilities, so the associations occupy an equally greater range. A soldier in the field can see in the far-off distance the dust rising from the approach of an enemy armored column. Though the danger is not yet immediate—certainly a snake would be given no cause for alarm—the association of the image is enough to elicit a brain stem response in the soldier. The cerebral interpretation of the situation creates the association of danger; the brain stem is informed, and physiological processes ensue.

The black-and-white nature of fight-or-flight can carry over into less-than-lethal scenarios. Since in most cases the interpretation of danger is funneled through the perceptive functions of higher parts of the brain, what the brain stem perceives as a threat to the organism can actually be a threat to the ego. This effect is seen in athletic competition. The combination of courage, determination, energy, and discipline an individual brings to athletic competition is often seen as representing the man himself; the collective character of the individual is held in the highest regard, to the point of sometimes superseding the actual physical ability of the individual or even the outcome of the contest itself. Harsh criticism awaits anyone who fails to put forth the greatest possible effort, and adulation for those who do. This, combined with the possible reward of winning—and therefore the realization of the sometimes supreme effort devoted to preparing for the event—is enough to alter the brain stem's interpretation of the event. Thus danger to the ego is perceived as danger to the organism. (Of course, many sports entail some physical danger, but there are few examples where the threat of death is very real. Big wave surfing is one.) Accordingly, athletic competition on occasion can precipitate a large adrenaline release.

The human brain stem carries the basic mechanical reasoning mechanisms of instinct. The brain stem is useful and necessary, but it isn't smart. It can be tricked. In the realm of athletic competition, the body is essentially being tricked into releasing adrenaline. Anticipation of the event itself—or components of the event, such as particular situations or plays—is enough to create that response. It is automatic. Thus can be the case with weight training. Anticipation of an extraordinarily grueling exercise can have the same effect, heavy barbell squats being an obvious example. This anticipation must be accompanied by supreme concentration.

Having elevated adrenaline levels has obvious benefits for weight training: More strength equals more intense muscular contractions, greater stimulation, and more growth. However, day-to-day weight training sessions have a much reduced ability to automatically spike adrenaline levels by themselves. Granted, more than a few people are able to show up at the gym, train very hard, and go home. For some, however, a mechanical switch for extremely hard physical work is not present. This is why some people will complain about a gym having a bad "atmosphere." For these individuals, brutal effort is not automatic, not a certainty; training next to others who are putting in a tremendous effort can be motivating. In the absence of added motivation, intensity levels can suffer and the workouts will therefore falter. So they are forced to look elsewhere, consciously or otherwise, for a boost. Sometimes the peripheral electricity of atmosphere cannot be found. Other external motivators must be identified, even if they come to exist only within the mind.

Within the mind there can be a real imperative to action; the ego can be threatened from within. A failure of the individual to live up to his own standards of courage, discipline, and determination should constitute a sufficient threat to the ego. Failure is failure, whether one is pitted against another or whether the competition is against one's own standards. If the sense of commitment to the task and self is strong enough, the lower brain can interpret this as a threat to the entire organism. With the most compelling associations, physiological processes will ensue, and the task can be met with a high level of energy.

A fundamental question raised by all of this is whether it can be possible to have high adrenaline production and Alpha brainwave activity simultaneously. Since Alpha brainwave studies all seem to center on intrinsically calm activities such as Zen, yoga, and sharpshooting, this is a matter of conjecture and deduction. It is doubtless that many weightlifters could offer anecdotes of having been in a state of adrenaline-aided motivation while at the same time possessing perfect concentration. But this combination can be seen regularly, one would surmise, by observing elite athletes. Those athletes experiencing the last few seconds before the gun in the finals of the 100-meter dash in the Olympics must have a combination of high adrenaline release and perfect concentration if they hope to prevail. Professional baseball on occasion also produces tense situations that are certain to raise adrenaline levels, yet there is an extremely high level of physical precision and therefore concentration required by that sport. Actually, all sports played at an elevated level have the potential for high-adrenaline situations that nevertheless require perfect concentration. So it seems that the answer must be yes.

Although a perceived "threat to ego" can actually help spike adrenaline levels, a significant increase should be considered rare. Such a spike will typically manifest itself when a particularly hard and heavy exercise, such as barbell squats, is about to get underway. A light isolation exercise such as dumbbell kickbacks won't elicit such a response, nor should it. Adrenaline release is reserved for dire circumstances and is always brief. Attempts to induce it should be economized. But for all exercises, and for the effort in its entirety, the unassailable commitment to task and self should be a primary motivating force. The ego is always threatened by failure, even if the circumstances do not create alarm great enough to alert the fight-or-flight mechanism. The ego is also rewarded by success, an equally strong motivator. The ability to avoid failure and achieve success is a product of determination.

Determination

Unassailable commitment to task and self cannot exist without sheer determination. Whereas obtaining the highest levels of energy possible can come about by riling the ancient brain stem, determination is a concept purely of the cerebral domain. It is in fact on occasion referred to as a "knightly" virtue. Determination within the context of weight training or athletic performance doesn't require much explanation. It drives the overall effort and insures that training sessions are optimal. Determination can also be seen as participating in the internal "threat to ego" struggle. A determined effort, carried through to success, gratifies the ego. An effort with insufficient determination is necessarily doomed.

Determination is perhaps the one intangible element that applies to all facets of a weight training campaign. Success in weight training far exceeds the mere act of lifting weights. A determination to succeed should include carefully choosing a viable strategy with particulars that will advance the campaign; another, more fiery version of determination will also be present at the moment of truth, when an all-out effort is getting underway.

In the most broad sense, since the military term of "campaign" has been used to describe a weight training plan, determination is the one thing that can ensure a realization of the end result—namely ultimate and final victory. "Ultimate and final victory" within the context of bodybuilding is actually the attainment of the desired level of development, maintained indefinitely. This is the whole point of the activity. Very few will undertake a campaign, for example, to gain 30 pounds of muscle, then quit training altogether, the desire having been satisfied. I have never known this to happen.

Gratification

But this ultimate and final victory is two-faceted, as part of it transcends mere body composition or strength goals; this particular portion of victory is gratification. The gratification of bodybuilding and fitness is the delayed type. True, there is a sense of well-being after a workout has been completed, but the real gratification takes place much further down the road. But once the gratification has been achieved, it can be maintained in a rolling fashion; it can be ongoing.

Intangible factors working in conjunction with a good, well-applied strategy, can contribute to the purpose of adding more muscle—which is after all the point of this book. But apart from completing his objectives, the weight trainer gets something else in return—and this might answer some questions regarding the motivation to build muscle, lift weights, or engage in any other type of strenuous exercise. Strenuous exercise is very gratifying.

Apart from the delayed but eventually ongoing gratification mentioned above, the emotional gratification of exercise seems to have two components, the first being of a directly physiological nature. Exercise triggers the release of the neurotransmitters seratonin and norepinephrine, two chemicals that provide a general sense of well-being and relaxation, and even pain relief. The second facet involves the satisfaction of having surmounted a difficult task, of putting forth a worthy effort and having accomplished something of no small measure. This can be experienced after a hard workout, or upon reflecting on the effort in its entirety. Accomplishment is gratifying. As the NFL coaching legend Vince Lombardi once remarked:

> "I firmly believe that any man's finest hour, his greatest fulfillment of all he holds dear, is the moment when he has worked his heart out in a good cause and lies exhausted on the field of battle—victorious."[30]

V

Conclusion

If you don't have a good plan, don't expect good results. This is an idea that transcends weightlifting, exercise, and even personal improvement in general. Really, it's an idea that applies to every field of human interest. It is a universal maxim. In bodybuilding, good results are something that everyone hopes for and many expect—but few are able to attain. Lack of a good overall plan is almost always the culprit. Nevertheless, there are individuals that hammer away at the weights, day-in, day-out for years. They do the same thing over and over but expect different results. Benjamin Franklin once wrote that such behavior defined insanity.[31] Modern psychiatric experts would doubtless have a more specific opinion on the definition of that word, but the point should be well taken.

Everyone thinks he has a good plan. Once in a while, after a period of dissatisfaction, some start to question their plans—a necessary first step towards improvement. Others hold fast in the face of dissatisfaction, deflecting blame from the true culprit, a poor plan. Consciously-held or otherwise, their training is based on an idea, and they are married to it.

One should never become married to an idea, lest he be prepared for the suffering of divorce. If he has unquestioning devotion to that idea, and it betrays him, what is he left with? Many are married to volume-oriented training; they fell in love quickly and settled into its routine, all because they have never known another. A small number flourish with this bride, and pay no mind to her imperfections, or never notice them. For many, she is a dreary and destructive burden, but somehow never forsaken, and never departed until the death of their training through mental or physical collapse. But for others, she turned out to be little more than a fling, or a foul mistress, cast aside once her imperfections were revealed.

I subscribe to the idea of high-intensity training. I can describe the theory behind it, and I use it—to good effect. But I am not married to it. I am ready to abandon it if its validity is trumped by the superior logic of another. Until that time, I will stick with it. It has a theoretical foundation, it works for me, and it consumes little time. It's satisfying, even fun. I don't think I could ask for a whole lot more. It is the cornerstone of my plan. I think it's a good plan, and I get good results, which I have the justification to expect.

Beyond this, it has kept me uninjured, no small accomplishment as I enter my twenty-fifth year of weight training. This point will be paid little attention by young ears, since the young have a tendency to think that their bodies are indestructible. When I was young, I thought so as well. As the years passed, I noticed the mounting casualty lists of dedicated weight trainers, people that I have known personally, and realized my training method was to thank as I stood unscathed. All the fallen were volume trainers. If there was just one point that I could make concerning the reasons for staying away from high-volume weightlifting, it would be the higher risk of injury. Train how you like, but keep in mind that the human body is *very* destructible. It is so destructible, in fact, that every single living being inevitably experiences total destruction.

High-intensity training has also allowed me to build a balanced physique. I am able to devote equal energy to all body parts, since I never wear myself ragged by performing a large number of sets for the first few exercises in a session. Many volume trainers perform double-splits to remedy this problem, but is such an approach something anyone would want or be able to sustain? And by now the point should have been well-taken that low-volume training is time-efficient. Having regular employment, I never would have had time to write this book had I spent all the extra hours in the gym as demanded by the volume approach. And who wants to spend all his free time in a gym?

I have precious few kind words for volume training. I have gone to lengths to describe its troubles, but ultimately volume training has fallen on its own sword. "God is dead" was metaphorically postulated by Friedrich Nietzsche in *Thus Spoke Zarathustra** as he challenged man to define his own morality when faced with the absence of religious direction. The religion of volume training was killed by Arthur Jones and Mike Mentzer, yet few are aware of this—as it to this day has a large following and remains the orthodox approach. High-intensity advocates

---

*The music bearing the same title ironically having been the bombastic overture of posing routines of many volume-trained bodybuilders during the 1980's.

metaphorically proclaim the death of that religion, and as such have been labeled by at least one supposed authority as "pagans." (And who would have thought weight-training theory might be analogous to nihilism?)

Volume training is inefficient. It is time and energy-consuming. At worst, it is totally ineffective and dangerous. It is not a sound investment. A few are able to get good returns from it, and they don't mind the time and energy demands, or the elevated risk of injury. Their approach is intuitive, their results plain to see. As thus, the method has a strong following—one that will never die. Thankfully, there is an alternative. But regardless of the type of training that one chooses to pursue, if he can logically justify employing his particular strategy, then he might well have a good plan. With such a plan in place, the results become a matter of hard training, consistency, proper nutrition, and of course genetic predisposition. Discussions of specific bad planning naturally gravitate towards volume training due to its distinct combination of rampant popularity and logical indefensibility.

The role of philosophy

There have been tremendous advances in the medical sciences over the past several hundred years, and the rate of important medical discovery is enjoying exponential progression. Nevertheless, much is still not known. In many ways the human body is what is known in technology circles as a "black box": Stimulus is fed to the body, and the response is noted. What actually takes place between the two events, within the black box, is often a mystery or at least unclear. If there was no mystery, and we already knew everything there is to know about the human body and how it operates, then there would be no need for medical research.

In the case of certain particular physiological functions, the way the human body operates and responds to stimulus is explained by theory, because there is not the absolute certainty of law. Theories are often constructed from hypotheses which have been arrived at through intuition or philosophical musing, or both. I don't know which specific process caused Hans Selye to formulate the general adaptation syndrome, but that mechanism is a philosophical physiological attribute, not a physical entity or organ. You can dissect a cadaver and easily locate and remove the heart, but you cannot extract and hold in your hand the general adaptation syndrome.

Selye's inspiration for the idea came about as a result of endocrinological studies on mice.[32] The details are not important, but what followed was a postulation on how the body generally responds to stress. Something about the observations suggested to him that a greater abstract mechanism was at work, and the theory was born. The idea was later applied to problem of the adaptation to stress of skeletal muscles. In this new context, empirical data confirmed that the idea held. And from this was created the theory of high-intensity training, a philosophically-conceived approach.

The existing lore of weight training methodology can be credited for coming reasonably close to reaching similar conclusions about the specifics of weight training through blind experimentation and hunches, but the prevailing ideas were always hamstrung by the intuitive more-is-better maxim. Actually, a more descriptive synopsis of the mindset behind what later became known as volume training is "the harder you work, the greater the returns—regardless of the specifics." For those who held, and for the masses that still hold this mindset, "harder" work almost always assumes the form of a greater volume of workload. It can be supposed that "the harder you work, the greater the returns" is also a philosophically-conceived dictum, though at a level that any and all can understand, and that few can resist.

One might try initiating a campaign to free the masses from the shackles of their logically bankrupt principles, but this will never work. "There's one born every minute," the phrase immortalized by W.C. Fields, applies perfectly to the endless stream of upstarts gripping a barbell for the first time. Almost none are aware that there is a science behind bodybuilding, few can define "science", and most never bother to consider what might be going on beneath the surface. Weightlifting is viewed as either a good, wholesome activity, or a vehicle to better health, more power, sexual attractiveness, or all of these things. As long as you're actually lifting weights, good things will follow, or so the mindset seems to suggest. I know, because a very long time ago I thought of it in a similar vein.

But alas, the road to hell is paved with good intentions. Volume training is a good intention, often carrying evil consequences. The words of the early twentieth century German military leader Hans Von Seeckt are worth revisiting: "Intellect without will is worthless. Will without intellect is dangerous."[33] A great number of weightlifters have will without intellect, if only because of their belief in the "hard work always pays off" mantra.

Intellect without will is a different story. Any lack of will among those who are regular gym-goers typically manifests itself as an unwillingness to produce absolute maximum effort during the actual workout. Of course, most weight training workouts enlist duration as a primary component at the cost of intensity, in which case the unwillingness actually becomes inability. A poor plan is the original cause, so the intellect is ultimately to blame—and in the end, if only within the context of the weight training environment, these hapless individuals can be observed to have neither intellect nor will. Countless gyms are filled with them.

In the face of poor physical results, a lot of these people nevertheless remain motivated to stick with the plan, and keep plodding along, all the while cursing their parents for having passed on inferior genes. They do not know that a reduced-volume strategy will allow for maximum intensity, since duration is not a factor—and that such an approach will create better results and therefore raise the basic level of motivation even higher. It is easy for me to get and remain motivated; I am in the gym less than four hours per week, and I am very happy with the results. But this happiness with results of course brings up one last and quite important question.

If the role of philosophy is to be considered within the arena of workout plan construction or performance optimization, it would be ignorant not to address a more fundamental philosophical question, that which was begged by the very first sentence of this book—anything worth doing is worth doing well—with the question of course being "is this something *worth doing?*"

Viewed from one perspective, the answer is an unqualified yes: Adding muscle mass increases athletic performance. Added size equals added strength. This extra strength means that one might run faster, jump higher, or hit a baseball farther. In football, the added mass alone will allow the player to deliver a greater blow with the body as he impacts another. Bodybuilding training, particularly the high-intensity variety, is perfectly suited for such increases in size and strength.

Bodybuilding proper, where the act of building muscle is the end purpose, is an entirely different matter. Those incapable of appreciating intellectual magnitude are naturally drawn to it, since everyone can appreciate physical magnitude, even lower animals. An intellectual justification is more elusive, and any rationalization must be more abstract. Inasmuch, it can be noted that the undertaking suits one criteria of Rand's Objectivism, as it can qualify as "productive achievement."[34] Since that particular philosophy also specifies that happiness is the moral purpose of life, pursuing a campaign of building mass is certainly worthwhile if the result is happiness. The happiness resulting from such a campaign can have several contributing factors, the first being the intangible satisfaction of achievement—that of the task itself, or of the achievement of aesthetic improvement, if this was one of the goals. The notion of aesthetic enhancement might cause some to misconstrue bodybuilding as a purely narcissistic endeavor. Narcissism has many forms—amassing great fortunes might be an exercise in narcissism for some—and those quick to point out the narcissism of bodybuilding might be unaware of these other forms, including those that they themselves might possess. (Granted, some bodybuilders are supremely narcissistic.)

But beyond the more abstract considerations, there are specific physiological mechanisms within the body that reward hard exercise. Hard exercise comes in many forms, weight training being just one flavor. But regardless of the type, optimum rewards always come from optimum execution. With all forms of exercise, this begins with having a good plan. The intellect thus has a role to play, that of outlining the strategy. The emotional being supplies the drive and motivation, and experiences the gratification of having properly executed the plan. Of course the body performs the physical execution, or stated more plainly, does the hard work, and ultimately, validates the effort in its entirety. But in the end the body need not be seen as all business—because, after all, it can also be said that the body gets to have all the fun.

Appendix A: Conan and the Wheel of Pain

Oddly enough, popular culture has had an inadvertent influence on the perpetuation of the volume training notion. It could not be more appropriate that the most famous volume-trainer of all time, Arnold Schwarzenegger, in a completely unintentional way helped to encourage the idea that endless hours of toil would create unusually great muscular growth. In his first major movie role as the title character in the Dino de Laurentiis classic *Conan the Barbarian*, a dramatic time-elapsed segment shows a pre-adolescent representation of Schwarzenegger shackled to the spoke of a giant revolving wheel, along with other boys of about his age. As the years pass, Conan continues to push the wheel around a never-ending circle, all the time gradually growing (in height and musculature) and surviving what is suggested to be the deaths of fellow prisoners. By the time he reaches adulthood, Conan—now played by Schwarzenegger—is the lone survivor. He is also massive. We are left to conclude that the laborious pushing of the wheel was the cause of this.

Of course, it was almost the duty of the filmmakers to offer *some* sort of explanation as to why Conan would have grown so large, so the Wheel of Pain was actually a pretty good idea. The concept was also able to adequately convey the idea that Conan was unbelievably tough. Who else could stand pushing the damn wheel around for 20 years? But despite the fact that *Conan the Barbarian* is a fantasy film with an abundance of supernatural elements, some people actually accepted the idea of the wheel, at a literal level, as a mass-building machine, or as a figurative representation of the notion that endless hours of brutal exercise will translate into massive growth.

The Friedrich Nietzsche quote that opens the film, "that which does not kill us makes us stronger" reinforces the deserted logic. In quite an ironic twist, the prevalence of misconception regarding the workload required for muscular growth can be adequately explained by another Nietzsche quote: "All things are subject to interpretation. Whichever interpretation prevails at a given time is a function of power and not truth."[35] The volume training idea has prevailed because of the power of the weight of opinion of those espousing it, the power of intellectual carelessness, and strangely, the odd pop culture snippet that draws upon the notion.

Be that as it may, I do feel that I have to point out that one aspect of the wheel idea as presented in the movie is correct: Conan was forced to endure progressive resistance. With the death of each of his wheel-pushing comrades, Conan had to work that much harder—until by the end he was pushing the wheel around all by himself. As we have seen, progressive resistance is one of the essential (and one of the few universally agreed-upon) principles of muscular growth. Unfortunately (or very fortunately, if you have ever seen that movie!) everything else with the wheel idea is wrong.

Appendix B: Anticipatory defense adaptation hypothesis

The stress-response mechanism of the Adaptation Principle is practical and straightforward. Beyond the practical specifics, a hypothetical mechanism of further defense might be at work. To shed light on this, it can be helpful to consider the vast array of mechanisms, sometimes quite novel, certain species have adopted to respond to or even anticipate the dangers of their environments.

Some of these attributes have an obvious function: Two forward-looking eyes provide stereoscopic vision and therefore depth perception. Predators tend to have this arrangement, since for them it is most important to focus on a single object, their prey. Even though the total time they actually have their eyes on a potential meal is probably very small, it is of utmost importance. The environmental danger for predators—natural enemies notwithstanding—is a lack of food. Go without it for long enough and the result is known to all. Conversely, eyes on the side of the head provide a large field of vision for herbivores, who usually have an abundance of food, but who also must be on the lookout for predators. Both are attributes that serve to preserve the animals that possess them, and indeed, the species themselves—so that they might eat or avoid being eaten.

Sometimes physiological or behavioral attributes can be far more subtle and even not apparent. The physiological reasons for our need to sleep are well-documented. But there might be other reasons as well. A few years back the interesting suggestion was made that sleeping can be a defense mechanism. For most mammals, sleeping keeps them quiet and low to the ground, which can be a somewhat effective passive defense mechanism. Maybe it was the case that nature began to favor animals— that through mutation required a certain amount of sleep for physiological repair—due to the success of this type of defense. To take it a step further, human snoring might have a similar, useful though now defunct reason for being. It might be more than the annoying design flaw we perceive it to be. Snoring, in purpose, might be a mechanism whereby a sleeping individual mimics a growling animal. A wandering predator might elect to bypass a group of snoring humans if they give the impression of being an angry, growling mob. One last example could be yawning. Contrary to popular belief, yawning is not caused by oxygen deprivation. In fact, research into the physiological benefits of yawning has proven inconclusive. But a reasonable theory is that yawning constitutes another passive defense mechanism, whereby the subject will periodically bare his fangs.

Muscles grow larger after they experience the stress of intense contractions. There exists a theoretically possibility that part of the mechanism that causes muscles to grow—namely, contractions of the highest possible intensity—might be the body's attempt to avoid fatal circumstances. To see what is meant by this, one might consider the prevailing notion that intense eccentric contractions, or negative repetitions, are of greater benefit than their positive counterpart. It seems logical that the body might be far more concerned with what it *cannot* do rather than what it can.

Negative reps, performed correctly (in a slow, deliberate manner) are, for all intents and purposes, failure. The body, though straining fiercely to accomplish the opposite, is unable to halt the descent of a weight. When performed with a great deal of intensity, this creates a significant impression on the muscle's physiological state. For all the body "knows," that particular furious muscular exercise, which in the end, despite all efforts, it was not able to overcome, had potentially fatal consequences. The body was faced with a task; it failed, and somehow the subject was able to escape with his life. It makes sense that the body would respond by trying to make itself better equipped, in the form of greater strength, to meet the challenge the next time around—so that it might prevail and preserve itself.

Assuming that this idea is true, then this bolsters the idea that negative reps are important, and furthermore: This is why it only takes a single set to stimulate growth. The challenge was met; despite a heroic effort, the subject failed. The message has been sent—period. The body knows it must adapt. *Now grow.* Subsequent sets are further damaging the muscle, but the stimulation has already been accomplished. Volume training is akin to sending the same message over and over. Other than the wasted time and energy, the idea of sending the same message repeatedly seems harmless enough, except that each time a message is sent, the messenger is worn down. With volume training, the damage will accumulate and will often become extensive enough that by the time of the next workout, the muscle and often the body itself will be in a state where it has not had sufficient time to fully repair itself and grow. In worse cases, it will not have had enough time to return to its state before the previous workout, and subject will actually be weaker—and this has all turned into an even bigger waste of time.

The idea of adaptation to stress is easy to fathom, but this poses a possible problem with the above-described life-or-death scenario: The idea assumes that the body knows when it is performing a negative rep—which it doesn't. The body *does* know, however, when a high-intensity muscular contraction is occurring. Since muscles are strongest during the eccentric phase of any repetition, with negative reps they can achieve the most intense contractions, making the greatest physiological impression on the body and therefore optimally stimulating growth. So for the purpose of stimulating muscular growth, negative reps *are* in fact of paramount importance due to the level of stress they are able to produce.

The fact that the body happens to be failing in its external task (resisting the object in the supposed life-or-death struggle) and is also performing a maximum muscular contraction might be coincidental, much as the passive-defensive nature of sleeping might be coincidental to the direct physiological benefits of that function. But the body need not directly equate maximum intensity contraction with external danger, much as it need not equate sleeping with achieving defilade from predators. In fact, the body doesn't "equate" anything. The mind does that. The body performs its functions, and the body responds to stimulus—and it belongs to a species that naturally and selectively adopts favorable characteristics. (The body doesn't "know" anything either; this word is used for lack of a better alternative.)

A point worthy of consideration is that a muscular contraction on the order of intensity required to achieve maximum stimulation (and therefore stimulate significant growth) in a prehistoric human should occur only in the most dire of circumstances. Prehistoric man did not lift weights, but he possessed the ability to grow large muscles nevertheless—and it's not hard to imagine that he would have sought to avoid all situations that would require any type of all-out effort. He was concerned with survival, not feats of strength and certainly not aesthetics.

It makes sense that stress of a life-or-death magnitude would then foster the most dramatic results—indeed, the degree of the body's response is in proportion to the intensity of whatever stress it encounters. This explains why non-weightlifting activities such as manual labor will often cause a slight increase in muscular mass among otherwise untrained subjects, and why the severe stress of high-intensity training can produce a dramatic increase in muscular mass. Additionally, for the purpose of achieving maximum physical productivity in a training session, it can actually help psychologically to imagine the task at hand as having life-or-death consequences. A more thorough investigation of the value of this association is alluded to in the *Intangibles* section

The idea of adopting a muscle-building response as a specific anticipatory defense mechanism is of course pure conjecture. However, its general action is hypothetically consistent with the general adaptation syndrome, which states that in the presence of a sufficient level of stress, the organism will perish.

Appendix C: Primary Instinctive Motivation

Mention was made in the *Intangibles* section of the role of human instinct. Humans possess ingrained behavioral attributes to aid them in the most important of their primary motivations, self-preservation. The purpose of the basic motivations for all creatures, especially this one, is perpetuation of the species. It is likely that over time species have existed with a different set of primary motivators, but of course the inferiority of their preservation mechanisms would have ensured their extinction. If a species cannot perpetuate itself, if it cannot insure its ongoing survival, then it will cease to exist. Indeed, all non-extinct species have successfully developed mechanisms to insure their survival. This does not mean that these attributes are necessarily beneficial to individual members of any species. The survival of any particular individual is of zero consequence (indeed, every last individual member will eventually die), as long as the species is able to avoid extinction.

All humans are guided by three primary instinctive motivators, though in general (and very interestingly) a discrepancy exists between the priorities of males and females. These motivators, in order of importance, are the following:

Males: Self-preservation, sex, and food.

Females: Self-preservation, food, and sex.

The idea of self-preservation topping the list for both sexes is easy to understand. A species has little hope of survival if its members do not place a priority on avoiding mortal danger or death. The following example illustrates the point: Gazelles will stop whatever they are doing, be it eating, resting, or mating, if a cheetah come running toward the herd. They will flee. Except perhaps for an unlucky example, they will all be saving their lives. They can resume their pre-stampede activities once the coast is clear.

But in order for a species to perpetuate itself, its members must breed, and they must eat. In other words, they must keep themselves alive, at least long enough to successfully breed, and they must replace themselves, since each and every individual will at some point die. Since males have a high level of motivation for sex, females have developed a de-prioritized attitude toward it. In general, males, seeking sex, find females and forthwith make sexual advances. Since males have made sex a high priority, there is no need for females do so, allowing eating to supersede it on the female priority list. In fact, some might argue that sex is not a primary motivating factor at all for females—except perhaps for certain lunarsynchronous or seasonal episodes.

Absent from the list is money, something that a great many people would cite as being one of their primary motivators. It is not. Money is recently-conceived entity, the possession of which being an avenue for the satisfaction of desires. It is not an inborn motivation, nor is it what drives creatures in the most fundamental sense. It can however be an instrument for placating the true primary motivating factors, and the cravings and fancies that derive from them. To lower animals who nevertheless share human instinctive motivations, it is of zero consequence. A cat will bat around a crumpled $100 bill for amusement, but will quickly abandon this game once he hears the sound of a can opener doing its bidding.

In the case of self-preservation, it has already been pointed out that instinct will tell humans to assume a sedentary posture at every possible turn. Some people gladly adhere to this request, and are purely sedentary. They do not ever willingly engage in any type of exercise. This mechanism developed when our existence required exercise—by gathering vegetation or hunting animals. As mentioned in the chapter on the Frequency Principle (p. 33), exercise requires rest. So our instinct tells us to get plenty of it. Nowadays, many humans can get by with doing nothing *but* resting. At the same time, rest is a necessary component of a good exercise regiment, so when the time comes, of course we should give in. And rest after hard exercise is the most satisfying type.

With food, humans have a biological mechanism that makes eating very pleasurable. This mechanism developed when food was scarce, so essentially the body wants us, when food is available, to eat as much as we can. In the twenty-first century Western world, food is available: Lots of it, all the time. And it's cheap. This, along with our instinct to remain sedentary, is why so many people are fat. Nowadays there are even fat homeless people.

Within the context of training purely for the purpose of gaining muscle mass, overeating is a non-issue. In fact, it's a little easier to put on muscle while eating very large amounts of food. However, pursuing a campaign to add muscle mass is very often born of a desire for aesthetic improvement. With this in mind, it is best to have a low level of body fat. Fat is not aesthetically pleasing. Despite what some would have us believe, the aesthetic ideal of the lean physique did not come about as a result of a brainwashing campaign from the media. Michelangelo was not brainwashed by the media when he created *David.* A fit physique (by this I do not necessarily mean a heavily-muscled bodybuilder, although some have this taste) is more sexually attractive. The impulse to overeat must be suppressed. At the same time, in a bodybuilding regiment it is most beneficial to eat frequently, though the meals should be relatively small and high in quality. In this respect the motivation to eat comes in handy, though again, the motivation must be managed and controlled.

This brings us to the other primary motivation, sex. For many, consideration of sexual desire caused them to realize that *if one is to be become fit and more sexually attractive, then the sexual urge can more easily be satisfied.* The process is rarely described in such plain terms, but this idea has been suggested in countless advertisements for diet or workout products, or gyms. The motivation for sex can be turned into a motivation to be in shape. Besides that, if the desire for sex is absent, would many people care if they were fat and sedentary? Many would not, but I tend to think that these people are not the types to devote their lives to exercise. And being in shape is certainly not the only avenue for increasing one's ability to satisfy sexual desire.

Beyond this and quite apart from any potential sexual motivations, hard exercise can be an avenue for various types of gratification. Of course, romantic relationships can be deeply emotionally gratifying as well—and perhaps being in shape can indirectly lead to a romantic relationship, in which case there is a sort of double emotional gratification. When enough emotional gratification is present, the result is happiness. At the same time, emotional gratification can come from a great many things, and indeed some happy people are neither fit nor in romantic relationships.

The desire to build muscle is also consistent with some of the human needs postulated by certain psychological theories. These ideas explain that much of human motivation and behavior originates from so-called psycho-sexual stages of development, including the need to be admired, the thirst for power, and even the inclination to be aggressive. The psychology behind bodybuilding or even immersion in exercise is itself a vast topic; entire books have been written on it. But it should be noted that the desire to build large muscles can have a complex foundation, and it can have a dignified execution and manifestation—and that in no way should it be misjudged as merely a crude ploy to get sex.

When addressing the specifics of instinctive motivating factors within the context of weight training or fitness in general, a workable strategy might include the ability to manipulate or manage certain motives (self-preservation and food) and the wherewithal to exploit the other (sexual desire). Clearly, this is not an approach propped up by piety or idealism. Doubtless some would find such a philosophy to be immoral. But given the biological hand that we humans have been dealt, it's practical. It is also consistent with Ayn Rand's Objectivism which declares that man's "own happiness (is) the moral purpose of his life, with productive achievement as his noblest activity, and reason as his only absolute."[36] Those claiming adherence to certain other philosophies or religions might find difficulty in justifying such an approach. And this brings up an interesting point: Who would have thought that bodybuilding or even training for fitness might pose a moral dilemma?

Notes

1. "Famous Self-Mastery Quotes," n.d., < http://www.thinkarete.com/ quotes/by_category/action/self-mastery/> (19 May 2007)
2. Paul Skinner, "Mike Mentzer: How Logic Forged a Vaid Theory," n.d., <http://www.mikementzer.com/skinnerlogic.html> (19 May 2007)
3. Mike Mentzer, "Heavy Duty, Chapter 1, Bodybuilders are Confused," n.d., <http://www.mikementzer.com/hdchap1.html> (19 May 2007
4. Selye, Hans. The general adaptation syndrome and the diseases of adaptation. Journal of Clinical Endocrinology 6:117-321, 1946.
5. A. Steinhaus, *The Journal of the Association for Physical and Mental Rehabilitation,* Vol. 9. No. 5, Sep-Oct, 1955, 147-150); W. Siebert and H, Petow, *Studien uberArbeitshypertrophie des Muskels,* Z. Klin Medl, 102, 427-433, 1925; Lange, Ueber Funktionelle Anpassung USW, Berlin, Julius Springer, 1917
6. Bryan Haycock, "Hypertrophy-Specific Training Q & A," October, 2001, <http://www.thinkmuscle.com/ARTICLES/haycock/hst-05.htm> (19 May 2007)
7. This summary of Mentzer's principles from Mentzer, Mike and Little, John R., *High Intensity Training the Mike Mentzer Way,* McGraw-Hill, 2002.
8. "Worlds in Collision," n.d., http://en.wikipedia.org/wiki/Worlds_in_Collision
9. Random House, 1979.
10. Fred Hatfield, "The Joe Weider Bodybuilding System," 2005, <http://www.musclenet.com/weiderbodybuildingsystem.htm> (19 May 2007)
11. *Ibid.*
12. "Microtrauma," n.d., <http://en.wikipedia.org/wiki/Microtrauma> (19 May 2007)
13. Mentzer, "Heavy Duty, Chapter 1, Bodybuilders are Confused," n.d., <http://www.mikementzer.com/hdchap1.html> (19 May 2007)
14. June 1997, < http://www.drweitz.com/scientific/injuries.htm> (19 May 2007

15. *Ibid.*
16. *Ibid.*
17. The American Journal of Sports Medicine 30:248-256 (2002)
18. "Overtraining," n.d., < http://en.wikipedia.org/wiki/Overtraining> (19 May 2007)
19. Haycock, "Hypertrophy-Specific Training Q & A," October, 2001, <http://www.thinkmuscle.com/ARTICLES/haycock/hst-05.htm> (19 May 2007)
20. *High Intensity Training the Mike Mentzer Way,* McGraw-Hill, 2002. p. 94-95.
21. *Ibid.*
22. Elizabeth Quinn, "Why Women are More Prone to ACL Injuries," February 2005, < http://sportsmedicine.about.com/od/kneepainandinjuries/a/women_acl.htm> (19 May 2007); "Sports Injuries," n.d., <http://www.pueblo.gsa.gov/cic_text/health/ sports/injuries.htm> (19 May 2007)
23. Currency, 1995.
24. *Ibid.*
25. "Ayn Rand," n.d., < http://en.wikipedia.org/wiki/Ayn_rand> (19 May 2007)
26. Walter Kaufman translation, part 13 of section 3.
27. "Flow (psychology)," n.d., <http://en.wikipedia.org/wiki/ Flow_%28psychology %29> (19 May 2007)
28. "Alpha Wave," n.d., < http://en.wikipedia.org/wiki/Alpha_wave> (19 May 2007)
29. "Beta Wave," n.d., <http://en.wikipedia.org/wiki/Beta_wave> (19 May 2007)
30. "Vince Lombardi Quotes," n.d., < http://thinkexist.com/quotes/vince_lombardi/> (19 May 2007)
31. "Benjamin Franklin Quotes," n.d., < http://thinkexist.com/quotes/ Benjamin_Franklin/> (19 May 2007)
32. "Hans Selye," n.d., <http://en.wikipedia.org/wiki/Hans_Selye> (19 May 2007)
33. Hans von Seeckt, *Thoughts of a Soldier*, trans. G. Water-house (London: Ernest Benn Ltd., 1930) p. 123.
34. Rand, Ayn. *Atlas Shrugged.* Signet Book; 35th Anniv edition, 1996.
35. "The Nietzsche Family Circus," n.d. < http://www.losanjealous.com/nfc/> (19 May 2007)

36. Rand, Ayn. *Atlas Shrugged.* Signet Book; 35th Anniv edition, 1996.

Index

Support Multiple Sclerosis research:

www.carantech.com   *Author photo by Dave Lepori.*